Stop
"Managing"
Diabetes...
Reverse it!

Naturally, safely and permanently

Alisa G. Cook, C.A., M.A.
Certified Traditional Naturopath

Forward by: Dr. Phyllis Cavanaugh

Other Books by the Alisa Cook:

Burn Fat, Build Muscle and Lose Weight in
Five Easy Steps.....Naturally and Permanently.
(co-authored with Dr. Phyllis J. Cavanaugh)

Forthcoming Book:

The GERD Cure

DEDICATION

To my parents, who believed in me as I embarked on this journey; and who taught me about eating fresh fruits and vegetables.

To Phyllis for your never ending support.

To my clients, past, current and future. We are on a learning journey, together.

To all the critters...

The saying, "You have everything if you have your health," is so true.

And, you can control more about that statement than you've been led to believe.

Believe...

Alisa G. Cook, CTN

Table of Contents

IMPORTANT NOTE

Throughout this book, several terms will be used to describe the disease of Type II Diabetes Mellitus, including, but not limited to:

- Type II Diabetes

- Type 2 Diabetes

- Diabetes

Under no circumstances should it be assumed that the author believes, or is suggesting, that Type I diabetes is curable at this time, although medical research toward that end continues and shows some promise.

Further, please note that individual results will vary. As long as a patient's pancreas is still producing insulin, there is a possibility that their condition of Type 2 diabetes is reversible. However, other factors may interfere, such as advanced organ system failure or other advanced disease complications. With that said, the program outlined in this book may still help the advanced Type 2 and Type I diabetes sufferer improve his or her quality of life.

ACKNOWLEDGMENTS

There are many natural health practitioners whose work I have studied, and whose approach to treating clients with the utmost of dignity and respect, I try to model. Some of them are well known in the field, and others are practitioners who I have seen on a personal health level.

Jeffrey Moss, DDS
Dicken Weatherby, ND
Phyllis Cavanaugh, DC
Jeffrey Bland, PhD
John Keifer, DC
Autumn Holder, ND
Andrew Weil, MD
Barry Sears, PhD
Scott Jamison, ND
Nancy M. Turcich, RPE
Daniel Kalish, DC

GLOSSARY

Diabetes: A variety of conditions that relate to blood sugar dysregulation. Patients with diabetes have an increased risk of heart disease, stroke, nerve damage, blindness and non-traumatic amputations, drastically reducing quality-of-life. Diabetes also has been shown to accelerate aging by facilitating an increase in cell damaging free radicals.[1]

Glucose: A simple sugar, also known as "blood sugar" fuels each of your approximately 60 trillion cells in your body. Primarily produced by the breakdown of carbohydrates during digestion.

Hemoglobin A1C: Also referred to as A1C, this is a measurement of your glucose, or blood sugar, over a three-month window. This bio marker is very important to track as it tells you how well you are managing blood sugars.

Hypoglycemia: A state in which blood sugar levels are too low.

Hyperglycemia: When blood sugar levels are too high.

Hyperinsulinemia: When insulin levels are too high, causing a wide variety of damage to the body.

---

1 Ceriello, Bortolotti, and Crescentini, "Antioxidant Defences Are Reduced During the Oral Glucose Tolerance Test in Normal and Noninsulin-dependent Diabetic Subjects."

Insulin: Produced by the beta cells of the pancreas, this hormone helps move glucose into your cells.

Insulin sensitivity (or insulin receptivity): This is the normal and ideal state in which your cells are sensitive to insulin's actions.

Insulin resistance: Elevated glucose levels, over time, trigger an increase in insulin levels. The insulin receptors on the body's cells eventually become "numb," or insensitive to the insulin, causing the glucose in the blood stream to rise, and the cells not receiving enough of the glucose fuel to operate optimally.

Ketoacidosis: Acidosis, caused by excessive production of ketone bodies due to a lack of insulin. Type 1 diabetics are more likely to develop this life-threatening condition, but it can also develop with Type 2, usually when the patient is severely ill.

FORWARD BY DR. PHYLLIS CAVANAUGH

Chronic Illness and Chronic Stress

This book is a radical departure from most of the diabetes books available on the market today. Instead of simply educating you about diabetes and how to "live with" or "manage" the disease that you have, this author has taken the bold step of telling you the truth. Diabetes is reversible! The concept that the body is a self-healing organism and that "disease" is most often not a pathological process at all but the body's attempt to adapt to a stressful, unhealthy environment, has been around for centuries. It is not, however, the basis of the traditional health care model that we are subjected to in this country.

In order to gain the most from this revolutionary book, we must begin to understand health in a different way. The traditional model of "health care" is not working. There is an avalanche of chronic illness in our country, indeed in most westernized societies, that is overwhelming us and, in order to deal with this new reality, it is essential to view your health in a different way.

The traditional health care model is not only inadequate in addressing the new reality of chronic illness, it does not generally acknowledge the true cause of illness and ultimately does not improve our health. If it did, we would be the healthiest nation on earth since we spend the most, by far, per capita.

Typically, a patient is examined, diagnosed with a disease, and a treatment protocol is started, usually involving medication. These medications are designed to suppress or stimulate symptoms so that you will "feel" better, but not necessarily be healthier. However, more and more people are being diagnosed with multiple illnesses. How many people do you know, for example, who have heart disease, diabetes AND thyroid problems? This approach to health breaks down very quickly as these multiple problems are "managed" with medications which quickly begin to cause problems themselves. The side effects from pharmaceuticals are a major source of emergency room visits. In fact, in 1998, The Journal of the American Medical Association reported an estimated 220,000 deaths are a result of properly prescribed medications - each year.

Although medical care has to be recognized for its very important ability to save lives in an emergency situation, deal with the life threatening disease of cancer, and for having developed amazing diagnostic tools that can assess the internal workings of your body to a minute degree, it is woefully inadequate as a means of addressing the chronic conditions facing our society today. We cannot continue to believe the fallacy that there is a prescription out there for every ill that comes our way, that if we could only fine-tune the diagnosis we could then find the correct prescription or combination of prescriptions that would "fix" us.

What if I told you that what is typically called "disease" is actually your body's attempt to respond to it's environment? Many of the most common health problems that we encounter today are actually your body's attempt to heal itself. Instead of looking at the health issues as "disease," we should, instead, look at them as "symptoms" and start to try to understand the underlying causes of these problems instead of trying to suppress them with medication. Please remember that pharmaceuticals suppress or stimulate but never heal. They do not cure a disease but suppress the major, unpleasant symptoms that manifest, thus allowing us to carry on with our lives without making the necessary changes to achieve true health. Health does not come in the form of a pill and disease is not caused by a deficiency of pharmaceuticals in our bodies; so why are we all taking so many drugs?

Let's step back for a moment and look at the big picture.

The body has an amazing ability to respond to its environment. When a stress affects the body, it responds in a time tested and predictable way, regardless of what the stress is. This response has been called the Stress Response, the General Adaption Syndrome, the Innate Intelligence and more. But the point to remember is that this response is the same for any stress, whether that stress is physical, emotional or chemical. Did you ever wonder why your heart beats faster when you think of something stressful? If you are laying awake at night worrying about paying the bills, your body senses danger and initiates the stress response. It's as if a saber toothed tiger is about to pounce on you.

The health problems that are facing many of us are a result of chronic stress response in our bodies that has gone on too long. It is as if the tiger is constantly chasing us but never quite catching us. Our society has become a very stressful place to live and our body responds in the only way it knows.

Let's take a closer look at the stress response to understand how it relates to this avalanche of chronic illness we are experiencing as a society. Remember, the physiological changes that are part of the stress response are the body's attempt to adapt to a change in its environment, whether that change is an actual tiger in the room, an emotional tiger or a toxic, chemical tiger.

The first thing that happens is that your nervous system senses danger and conveys that to your brain; Danger! The fight or flight response is initiated and it is powerful, overriding many of the body's mundane processes to prepare us for "battle." The sympathetic nervous system is the alarm system that sets many of these processes in motion and sends them out to all systems in the body.

The adrenal gland is stimulated to release hormones which act on the heart to increase the heart rate and the stroke volume while at the same time causing vaso-constriction of the blood vessels going to the organs of digestion. These factors allow for rapid delivery of the stress hormones to all the systems of the body and also allows the muscle easier access to the blood sugar that starts pouring into the blood from storage.

In fact, the body prepares for a battle by releasing triglycerides as well as glucose into the blood stream. Over time, as the stores are depleted, the body will often break down muscle tissue (protein) and convert it into glucose, resulting in a loss of muscle mass. There is also an increase in blood cholesterol as it is needed for the steroid based stress hormones as well as for potential wound healing. The stress response also increases clotting factors for the same reason.

The increase in blood glucose causes an increase in insulin. At the same time cortisol (an adrenaline hormone) results in a down regulation of insulin receptors. This makes sense as the body is in "break-down mode" (pull energy into the blood for use) instead of "building mode," which is what insulin stimulates So, glucose and insulin are both elevated with an increased insensitivity to insulin at the cellular level. Over time, this can result in insulin insensitivity, the precursor of diabetes.

The stress response also activates the parts of the brain that relate to anxiety and stress and decreases the ability to sleep and to concentrate. We do not need to be able to learn if a tiger is chasing us.

Remember, the stress response is designed for a short-term, emergency situation and is extremely effective in saving your life. It begins to cause serious problems when the stress never ends and the body continues to attempt to adapt to an unhealthy environment. Let's look at the results of a chronic stress situation that goes on too long.

- Adrenaline and Cortisol levels are elevated

- Increased heart rate
- Increased blood pressure
- Increased blood sugar
- Increased triglycerides and cholesterol
- Muscle mass is lost
- Clotting factors are increased
- Serotonin levels are decreased
- Sensory and pain receptors are sensitized
- Increased anxiety and depression
- Decreased memory and concentration
- Decreased sex hormones
- Decreased bone density

These are the precursors of all the major illnesses in our society: heart disease, stroke, cancer, diabetes, depression, sexual dysfunction, osteoporosis and more; and these are all, for the most part, preventable and reversible diseases.

The solution is not to take a pill to suppress the symptoms, but rather to change the factors that are causing the chronic stress in the first place. This is the problem we face; there is no magic pill (pharmaceutical, natural or otherwise). We have to do the work of looking at our lives to see where we are continuing the cycle of chronic stress and work to break it.

Alisa Cook's ground breaking book, "Stop Managing Diabetes...Reverse It!" takes an honest look at the stress put on our bodies by an unhealthy, unnatural diet of high carbohydrates and the devastation of type 2 diabetes that results. She lays out the process of reversing diabetes, step by step. After reading this book, you will look at your food and your health in a totally different way. All of the symptoms that you have been living with will start to make sense. They are all part of a process, an attempt by the body to adapt to an unnatural environment; not isolated, unrelated events. When you start the process of removing the obstacles to allowing the body to heal and return to balance, you will begin to notice not just an improvement in your blood sugar levels, but in all aspects of your health.

Enjoy the journey!

Dr. Phyllis Jean Cavanaugh
Bisbee, Arizona
September, 2012

drc@bisbeechiropractic.com

INTRODUCTION:
THE POTENTIAL OF OPTIMAL HEALTH

"Health is a state of complete physical, mental and social well-being and not merely the absence of disease or infirmity."

World Health Organization

You may have picked up this book because you have been diagnosed with diabetes, or you've been told that you're pre-diabetic. Perhaps you're reading it because you have a loved one in your life who is suffering from diabetes. Or, maybe you're reading it because you are trying to avoid diabetes in the first place.

Whatever the reason, this book is written to help you either prevent or reverse the disease, and do something even more important; help you create a life of optimal health vs. one that is just free of disease.

Optimal Health vs. "Health"

The notion of optimal health is not a new one, especially within the realm of natural health. I will have done my job as a writer of this book if I help you not only reverse a destructive disease process, but also help you achieve what I call optimal health.

Too often in our society, we think of health as an absence of disease. In other words, as long as you don't have a disease or "condition" applied to you, you are healthy. To some extent, I suppose, this is true. But, there is quite a difference between feeling optimally healthy and being "healthy" by merely being free of disease.

I have met with many clients in my practice who, by conventional medicine standards, are "healthy." Their blood work values are "normal," and any other tests that may have been run are "normal." However, the client is seeing their physician because something is wrong. Maybe they're tired all the time, or they've noticed muscle weakness. Perhaps they're gaining weight and are having a hard time losing it. Maybe they've noticed that their skin and hair are more and more dry and brittle. Possibly they're going to see the doctor because they've noticed their heart racing and they're prone to heavier sweating. They're worried. But, since all tests are "normal," they're sent home with no reassurances or real assistance otherwise.

The above symptoms, however, aren't normal, and something is wrong. The patient doesn't feel well; he or she is struggling to get through the days and is no longer doing things that he or she loves to do. Maybe you can see yourself in this description; maybe you feel tired all the time, you just don't have the energy that you used to. Your joints are getting stiffer and more inflamed, and you have chronic pain. Maybe you've chalked it up to "growing old." I'm here to tell you that you don't need to live that way.

Optimal health is very, very different from the above scenario. When you are optimally healthy, you feel great. You have more energy than you thought possible at your age. You feel hopeful and optimistic about your future health, and you are enjoying getting older, instead of dreading the next week, month, or year of feeling less than good. When you are optimally healthy, you are not only free of serious diseases, you feel younger than you did before you started on this pathway toward optimal health.

So, before we get too far in this book, know that this is my "hidden agenda." I don't just want you to prevent or reverse a terrible disease. I don't just want you to reduce your dependency on harmful pharmaceuticals. I want you to finish with your wellness program that we will describe in this book and say to yourself, your friends, your colleagues, your family members, "I feel great! I can't believe it!"

That is my wish for you. Before we even discuss the disease process of diabetes, and how you can reverse it, I want you to know that optimal health is a possibility for you; what you are able to achieve will be different than the next person, but *your* level of optimal health is achievable.

This is not just a book about striking the word diabetes from your personal vocabulary, this is a book about how to feel great.

The Importance of Working with a Diabetes Counselor

Though this book will give you the background information on how to reverse diabetes, including dietary information, stress relief tips, exercise ideas, and much more, it is not enough.

I have seen too many people start and fail an endeavor like you are about to undertake. They go into it with the best of intentions, and with a true commitment to change their lives. But, after a few months, usually two or three, they lose steam and they start to see their progress slow down, and eventually get frustrated and give up. This is a marathon and not a sprint, and you need support.

Imagine the marathon runner trying to make it without any outside support. No one to hand them a refreshing cup of water, no one to cheer them on, and no one to boost them up when they're feeling like they can't go on any further.

You, dear reader, are on a marathon run, and you need the type of support that only an experienced and knowledgeable diabetes counselor can provide. You need someone to hold you accountable, and to "make you" show up; show up to regular meetings *(at least* twice monthly), and show up emotionally and spiritually for the journey that you are about to embark on.

I am not stating this based merely on my own personal experience, nor just on my experience as a natural health practitioner. This is a fact that has been articulated in the medical literature for decades. One recent landmark study, which I will discuss in further detail later, published in the *Diabetes Care* journal of the American Diabetes Association, is an excellent example of this assertion.

A meta-analysis of over 30,000 patients who were diabetic, this study examined success rates, and the time it took to be successful, depending on whether or not the patient participated in a comprehensive wellness program where they met with an experienced counselor more than once a month, or if they merely went in for checkups with their doctor every 6 months or so.

The results were interesting, to say the least, and can be life changing, for you...

Those that participated in the comprehensive wellness program reached their goals (blood glucose, blood pressure, A1C, etc.) within 5-6 months. Those that went it alone, *if* they reached their goals, did it within 22-25 months.[2]

How soon do *you* want to see results. Do you want to celebrate your successes before your next 6-month checkup with your doctor? Imagine his or her surprise when your blood work is being reviewed and the evidence of all your hard work is clearly evident.

---

2   Morrison, Shubina, and Turchin, "Lifestyle Counseling in Routine Care and Long-Term Glucose, Blood Pressure, and Cholesterol Control in Patients With Diabetes."`

Two quick success stories for you to consider (you are not alone in this process, and you will not be alone in your success).

Richard came to my office after being diagnosed with diabetes several years prior. We worked together, long-distance (he in New York state, me in Arizona), initiating changes in his diet, exercise routine, and stress management. After conducting a thorough medical history, I also recommended a few key supplements that are designed to help reverse insulin resistance and the diabetic process. We met twice a month, via phone meetings, and emails in between visits.

Four months after starting the program, Richard went to his regular doctor, who exclaimed, upon reviewing the blood work, "Oh my God....you're reversing your diabetes. I don't see this very often."

Linda, a gentle soul of a client, also diagnosed with diabetes, though more recently, has, at this writing, worked with me for just three months. In that time, she reports that her fasting glucose, with oral hypoglycemic medications, has dropped from an average of 230 to 97-120. We have a long way to get to optimal (75-86), but we are both highly encouraged by her initial progress. Her ultimate desire is to shed her need for medications, and reverse her disease naturally. I have no doubt that she will achieve her goals.

Who should you work with?

There are several types of counselors that you can work with. Certified Diabetes Educators in your community may have programs, or you can work with a natural health practitioner who has experience helping people reverse insulin resistance and diabetes.

The most important criteria, beyond proven results, is the feeling of trust and connection that you must have with your diabetes counselor. He or she will become a vital member of your diabetes support team (which includes your physician, endocrinologist, podiatrist, optometrist, etc.) You must feel that you can confide in this person your concerns, your struggles, your fears. The relationship that you have with your diabetes counselor can literally help you change your life forever.

The American Diabetes Association will tell you to only work with Certified Diabetes Educators. I disagree. I have met many practitioners who are highly qualified and experienced in this regard. My preference, of course, is that you also work with someone who understands the natural health realm and who designs comprehensive, individualized programs that are based on scientific research.

It's also important to make sure that, whoever you work with, understands the physiology behind the disease; what is going on to create the malady, and specifically and exactly how to customize a program that will work for you.

If I can help in any way, please feel free to contact me. My job is to help you learn about how to reverse this disease, and to make sure you have the support that you will need.

Alisa G. Cook, C.A., M.A., C.L.E.
Certified Traditional Naturopath
520-366-1646
gaiawellness@ymail.com
http://www.facebook.com/gaiawellness

WHAT IS DIABETES,
AND HOW DID YOU GET HERE?

*I am the only person in the world I
should like to know thoroughly.*

Oscar Wilde

First of all, I don't want to imply that your having
diabetes is your fault. We all do the best we can with
what we know, and things happen to us that, at least
initially, we don't have any control over. If you have
made mistakes in the past, it may be because you didn't
know any better. Or, perhaps you did, and now that
you're older, and wiser, you realize that you want to walk
a healthier road.

When I meet with clients, more often than not I am
sharing with them new information that they did not
know and/or haven't heard from their doctor. By taking
the time to go over the details of what we know about

type 2 diabetes, the physiological and pathological processes in place, we can better understand the reversal process. (What better way to reverse course than to understand how you got where you are in the first place?)

So, what is diabetes, anyway?

Simply stated, diabetes is when the body either does not produce enough insulin (the hormone that helps glucose, fuel for every cell, get up-taken by the cells), or the effect of insulin is reduced due to cellular damage from consistently excessive insulin released by the pancreas in response to a high sugar diet.

The result is excess insulin, as well as high glucose or sugar levels in the bloodstream, leading to hyperglycemia (high blood sugar). This can ultimately lead to very serious short- and long-term adverse health effects including kidney failure, heart disease, elevated cholesterol and triglycerides, permanent eye damage, neuropathy or damage of the nerves in the feet and/or hands, and much more.

Types of diabetes

There are several types of diabetes that you may have heard of: type 1 diabetes mellitus (formerly identified as juvenile diabetes or insulin dependent), type 2 diabetes mellitus (formerly known as adult-onset diabetes, or non-insulin dependent), gestational diabetes, and diabetes insipidus (more related to the kidneys' function than the kind of diabetes that we will be discussing in this book).

Type I Diabetes Mellitus

Many (approximately 25-30%) diagnoses of type 1 diabetes mellitus occur when an individual is experiencing some degree of diabetic ketoacidosis (DKA)[3], a severe complication which, if left untreated, eventually results in diabetic coma and death. Initial symptoms include intense thirst, excessive urination, extreme hunger, unusual weight loss and a state of exhaustion and severe fatigue.[4]

With type 1 diabetes, the beta cells of the pancreas are not producing enough insulin, or the insulin produced is defective. These patients always require external sources of insulin and self-control of blood sugar levels to avoid serious complications.

The cause of type 1 diabetes is thought to be an auto-immune destruction of the beta cells in the pancreas. What causes the auto-immune response is currently being studied, with the primary suspect being a severe emotional or physical trauma, a virus, or other chronic physical stress and/or systemic inflammation.[5] There is also a very strong genetic component to acquiring type 1 diabetes.

---

3 Lilley, Harrington, and Snyder, *Pharmacology and the nursing process.*

4 "Symptoms - American Diabetes Association."

5 Lilley, Harrington, and Snyder, *Pharmacology and the nursing process.*

Type 1 diabetes mellitus is relatively rare, constituting only 5% of all diabetes diagnoses.[6]

Type 2 Diabetes Mellitus

Long thought to be a mild form of type 1 diabetes, type 2 diabetes is by far the most common, accounting for approximately 95% of all diagnoses.[7] There are many common and dangerous misunderstandings about type 2 diabetes:

- That it is a mild form of diabetes
- That it is easy to treat
- That tight blood sugar regulation is not necessary, because the medications will "take care of it"

Type 2 diabetes is due to either (or sometimes both) insulin resistance (see *The Insulin Trap* chapter for more detailed information) or an insulin deficiency. A way to think of insulin resistance is that the receptors on your cells are becoming "calloused" due to over stimulation; like when a new guitar player develops calloses on his or her fingertips, which cause the fingertips to become a bit numb.

Just as your cells, over time, may become insensitive to insulin, creating insulin resistance, the beta cells of the pancreas can become insensitive to the presence of glucose, resulting in a type of glucose insensitivity.[8] This

---

6   "Type 1 - American Diabetes Association."

7   American Diabetes Association, "Where Do I Begin? Living with Type 2 Diabetes."

8   Lilley, Harrington, and Snyder, *Pharmacology and the*

occurs because the beta cells, like the insulin receptors on each cell, become 'calloused' or 'numb' to the presence of glucose.[9] The result is a lowered production of insulin.

The good news is, and what this book is about, you can reverse insulin resistance and the glucose resistance, increasing insulin sensitivity and increasing the efficiency of the beta cells of the pancreas. Your body has an amazing capacity to heal itself.

There are several symptoms of type 2 diabetes, including all of those as outlined for type 1 diabetes. Additional symptoms include[10]:

- Frequent infections
- Blurred vision
- Tingling/numbness in the hands/feet
- Frequent and recurring skin, gum and bladder infections
- Cuts and bruises that are very slow to heal

However, it's important to note that there are millions of undiagnosed cases of type 2 diabetes (approximately 7 million, according to the American Diabetes Association)[11] as many cases of diabetes involve no symptoms. In fact, there are more people with pre-diabetes (at high risk for developing type 2 diabetes),

nursing process.

9 "Symptoms - American Diabetes Association."

10 "Diabetes Statistics - American Diabetes Association."

11 Ibid.

approximately 79 million, than with already developed diabetes (approximately 26 million).[12]

Gestational Diabetes

Occurring during pregnancy, gestational diabetes develops in about 2% of pregnancies.[13] Insulin is often prescribed to decrease the risk of birth defects. In most cases, the glucose intolerance of gestational diabetes subsides naturally after delivery of the infant. However, as many as 30% of women who developed gestational diabetes develop type 2 diabetes within 10 to 15 years of the pregnancy.[14]

Some scary statistics

Here is a summary of the status of diabetes in our country, according to the American Diabetes Association[15]. As you can see, we have a big problem here.

- As of 2011, there are 25.8 million people diagnosed with diabetes (both type 1 and type 2)
- Of those, 7 million are undiagnosed
- Approximately 8.3% of the U.S. Population has diabetes

12 "Diabetes Statistics - American Diabetes Association."

13 Lilley, Harrington, and Snyder, *Pharmacology and the nursing process.*

14 "Diabetes Statistics - American Diabetes Association."

15 "Diabetes Statistics - American Diabetes Association."

- More than 25% of the U.S. population has pre-diabetes, or insulin resistance, putting them at very high risk of developing type 2 diabetes
- If you add total diabetes cases and pre-diabetes, more than 30% of the U.S. population is either at high risk of developing type 2 diabetes, or has it already.
- Adults with diabetes have 2-4 times higher heart disease related deaths than non-diabetics
- Diabetes is the leading cause of new cases of blindness for ages 20-74
- Diabetes is the leading cause of kidney failure
- More than 60% of non traumatic amputations are caused by diabetes complications
- In 2007, costs related to diabetes were upwards of $217 billion
- The diabetic patient has health care costs that are 2.3 times higher than the non-diabetic

I learned long ago that these types of numbers don't motivate people, myself included. Let's face it, if good health numbers (blood pressure, glucose, cholesterol, etc.) truly motivated us, we would all be naturally healthy.

The truth is more personal. What motivates us to want to be healthy is usually because of how we feel, not scary statistics and almost meaningless numbers. What motivates us is wanting to do what we aren't able to do anymore. Things I've heard from my clients are statements like, "I want to have the energy again to do the things I love," or "I'm just sick and tired of feeling sick and tired."

So, let's leave the statistics behind, and move on to learn a little more about this "dis-ease" we call diabetes, and how you got here.

A (very) short history of diabetes

Diabetes mellitus has been identified for almost 5,000 years. The Egyptians described a malady that they called *honeyed urine*.[16] In 1788, an English physician named Thomas Cawley, published his opinion that the disease involved the pancreas.[17] It would take more than a century to prove this, and even longer to discover that the disease involved insulin, and that insulin was secreted by the pancreas. In fact, insulin wasn't isolated until the early 1920s[18] and its discovery is considered one of the greatest victories of 20th century medicine. Its use as a therapy for type 1 diabetes has been a life saver for millions of people over time.

But how did I get here?

Here's how it usually happens, but this may not be your specific journey to diabetes. Even so, it's likely that you followed this general progression of the development of type 2 diabetes.

- Sugar comes in many forms, some healthy and some definitely not. Either way, if you have an excess of sugars in all its forms in your diet, your pancreas will work overtime to produce the

16 Ibid.

17 Ibid.

18 Ibid.

insulin needed to reduce blood sugar levels in the bloodstream and increase cellular uptake of glucose.

- In time, your body becomes insensitive to insulin, and production of insulin becomes completely independent of actual demand; that is, the pancreas overproduces insulin because it's used to excess sugar in the blood, so even when blood sugars are low or normal, the pancreas will work extra hard to produce too much insulin (see *The Insulin Trap* for more detail).

- In the meantime, excess insulin triggers the body to store fat, causing weight gain and making it very hard to lose weight. You develop belly fat, and even if you're hungry, that fat won't be released because the insulin is telling the fat to stay there. (see "The Insulin Trap" chapter for more detail)

- As the process continues, the pancreas starts getting tired, and, eventually wears down prematurely, causing the reduction of insulin production. This can be further accelerated by oral hypoglycemics that stimulate the pancreas to produce more insulin (more on that later – see *The Myth of "Managing" Diabetes)*.

Now for the good news!

This chapter has been, admittedly, mostly a bad-news kind of report. But, I will end it with good news – no, exceptional news.

The process described above is reversible. Even if you've been walking on the path toward diabetes for some time, chances are you can now walk backwards and reverse this process. You can get to the point where you are at a new fork in the road; where you decide the route to optimal health, and you go down that road instead.

It's not an easy process, and it takes time, but you can reclaim your health and wellness. And, with the help of an experienced health counselor, and with regular visits and updates (more than once a month), you can accelerate your progress, reversing the primary signs (elevated glucose, elevated Hemoglobin A1C, elevated fasting insulin) in just 5 months (versus more than two years by going it alone).[19]

But, the bottom line is this....if you want it, you can have it. You can leave your diabetes in the dust!

---

19 Morrison, Shubina, and Turchin, "Lifestyle Counseling in Routine Care and Long-Term Glucose, Blood Pressure, and Cholesterol Control in Patients With Diabetes."

Alisa G. Cook, CTN

WHAT THE MEDICAL RESEARCH SHOWS ABOUT REVERSING INSULIN RESISTANCE AND DIABETES

*Somewhere, something incredible is
waiting to be known.*

Carl Sagan

I am a research-driven practitioner; many natural health providers do an injustice to the field, and more importantly to their clients, by relying on techniques and protocols with little or no evidence of their effectiveness. Some clients express nervousness that I might be yet another "woo woo," or "new age," practitioner when they first meet with me. This could not be further from the truth; though I do firmly believe in the power of the mind

to direct healing, and the importance of addressing
emotional and spiritual wellness when embarking on a
journey of optimal health, I am also a firm believer in
emphasizing wellness programs that have their foothold
in research.

This chapter is placed toward the beginning of the book
for several reasons. First, the notion of reversing type 2
diabetes is not just a "nice idea," as a client said to me
once, not quite convinced that her disease was something
she could, indeed, reverse. It is something that is well
documented, and has been for several decades. Second,
rather than get bogged down in citing research throughout
the book, I aim to offer the reader a one-stop-shop to
peruse current research on this topic, organized into
categories that make sense. Finally, the links to accessing
the full research articles (available on the companion
website www.stopmanaging.diabetes.com) are included
so that you can review the primary source, and not just
my interpretation.

> Increasingly, scientific and medical articles...and
> commentaries...about diabetes interventions use the
> terms "remission" and "cure" as possible outcomes.
>
> American Diabetes Association
>
> Buse et al., "How Do We Define Cure of Diabetes?".

The above quote is taken from a recent consensus statement of the American Diabetes Association, where the authors agreed that complete "remission" of the disease of type 2 diabetes could be attained when normal measures of glucose metabolism are measured for over one year, and without pharmaceutical intervention.[20] So, this idea of reversing, or curing, diabetes is not a unique one that I have decided to proselytize about; it is, rather, a well established reality that, for some reason, the conventional medical establishment has not passed along to diabetic patients. For evidence of this, consider a quote from a publication called, "Getting Started With Diabetes," by the American Diabetes Association:

"There is no cure for type 2 diabetes, but it can be managed."[21]

More often than not, when I mention the reversibility of Type 2 diabetes to clients or potential clients, they respond with a statement like, "How come my doctor has never told me that?" To that question, I don't have an answer. The important fact remains that, for the vast majority of diabetic patients, their disease is reversible and, in fact, curable, even if it has progressed to the point that the patient is injecting themselves with insulin.

20 Buse ct al., "How Do We Define Cure of Diabetes?".

21 "Getting Started With Diabetes - American Diabetes Association."

This is not a comprehensive list of the research supporting the reversibility of type 2 diabetes. I have hand selected certain articles that drive the point home, and have only selected articles from highly respected peer-reviewed journals like *Diabetes Care* by the American Diabetes Association, and the *Journal of the American Medical Association*.

These research articles are categorized as follows:

- Reversing Signs and Symptoms of Diabetes and Insulin Resistance

- Reducing Risk/Preventing the Disease

- The Importance of Counseling/Coaching

Category 1: Reversing Signs and Symptoms of Diabetes

There are a myriad of symptoms of Type 2 Diabetes, including:

- Increased thirst and urination

- Unexplained weight loss or weight gain

- Fatigue/tiredness

- Increased hunger, even after eating

- Shakiness in between meals

- Headaches

- Slow healing of cuts and/or sores

- Numbness and tingling of hands and feet

Most individuals who are diagnosed with Type 2 Diabetes don't even know that they have the disease, and only upon hindsight do they take note of the above symptoms. More often than not, diabetes is diagnosed based on the signs of the disease, primarily through blood work.

- Hemoglobin A1C is 6.5% or higher

- Fasting blood sugar level is 126 mg/dL or higher

- Oral glucose tolerance test is 200 mt/dL or higher

- Random blood sugar level of 200 mg/dL or higher (along with the symptoms of high or low blood sugar)

Clustering of Multiple Healthy Lifestyle Habits and Health-Related Quality of Life Among U.S. Adults With Diabetes[22]

---

22 Li et al., "Clustering of Multiple Healthy Lifestyle Habits and Health-Related Quality of Life Among U.S. Adults With Diabetes."

One of my favorite medical research articles refers specifically to the quality-of-life of patients with diabetes. Numbers are numbers (e.g. glucose, A1C, insulin levels), but the most important factor when we think of health is, "How do I feel?" If good numbers truly motivated us, healthy cholesterol levels, blood pressure, etc., we would all be healthy. But, the truth is, we are rarely, if ever, motivated to "lower our numbers," as much as we are motivated by the desire to live a longer, healthier life where we have the energy to do the things we love to do.

This particular research article explored this notion, along with some of the numbers that are tied to being classified as a diabetic. First, the authors identified four Health Related Quality of Life (HRQOL) factors; general health rating, physically unhealthy days, mentally unhealthy days and impaired activity days. The authors then identified three Healthy Lifestyle Habits (HLH); not smoking, participating in adequate physical activity, and consuming five or more servings of fruits and vegetables.

Their conclusion was that when a patient consistently instituted a variety of healthy lifestyle habits, their quality of life significantly improved. They felt better; experiencing less symptoms than their counterparts that didn't partake in healthy lifestyle habits.

Biologic and Quality-of-Life Outcomes From the Mediterranean Lifestyle Program; A randomized clinical trial[23]

Another study on quality of life, as well as some of the measurable aspects of diabetes (glucose, A1C, etc.), here the authors explored the effectiveness of a comprehensive approach to diabetes management using, what they called a Mediterranean Lifestyle Program (low saturated fat Mediterranean diet, stress management training, exercise, support, and smoking cessation.) The subjects of this study were post menopausal women with diagnosed type 2 diabetes. Participants took part in a 3-day retreat, followed by six months of weekly follow-up meetings.

Significant reductions and normalization in A1C, lipids (cholesterol, LDL, HDL, triglycerides), blood pressure, plasma fatty acids and increased flexibility were noted. Additionally, participants noted a significant improvement in their stated quality of life.

Effect of Calorie Restriction With or Without Exercise on Insulin Sensitivity, β-Cell Function, Fat Cell Size, and Ectopic Lipid in Overweight Subjects[24]

---

23 Toobert et al., "Biologic and Quality-of-Life Outcomes From the Mediterranean Lifestyle Program."

24 Larson-Meyer, "Effect of Calorie Restriction With or Without Exercise on Insulin Sensitivity, -Cell Function, Fat Cell Size, and Ectopic Lipid in Overweight Subjects."

In this study, the authors examined the possibility of
reversing insulin resistance (the primary cause of
diabetes) by caloric reduction, exercise or both. They
found that insulin resistance could be reversed with either
caloric restriction or exercise, adding that the sensitivity
to insulin increased with a reduction in weight, fat mass
and visceral fat (fat located in and around the organs –
behind the abdominal muscle wall).

*Lifestyle Changes May Reverse Development of the
Insulin Resistance Syndrome. The Oslo Diet and Exercise
Study: a randomized trial*[25]

I've included this study, even though it is quite a few
years old (1997), to point out that the reversal of insulin
resistance, the primary cause of diabetes, is not a newly
discovered possibility. In this landmark study, the
researchers wanted to, "compare and assess the single and
joint effect of diet and exercise intervention for 1 year on
insulin resistance and the development leading toward the
insulin resistance syndrome."[26]

In this study, the authors selected 219 men and women
who did not have diabetes, but who had measurable

---

25 Torjesen et al., "Lifestyle Changes May Reverse
  Development of the Insulin Resistance Syndrome. The Oslo
  Diet and Exercise Study."

26 Ibid.

insulin resistance (the second step toward the disease progression of diabetes, the first being reactive hypoglycemia). After one year of either dictary changes, diet and exercise, exercise only, or no changes, any correlating changes were noted. In the diet-only group, significant reductions in insulin resistance were noted, with even greater reductions in the diet and exercise group. According to this study, exercise alone did not result in improved insulin sensitivity.

Category 2: Reducing Risk/Preventing the Disease

Diabetes comes with its fair share of health risks; unfortunately, diabetics can count on a shortened life, and a much lower quality of life, if they do not take control of the disease, and kick it out of their life, forever. Many of the risks are well known, including:

- Nerve damage, especially to the feet, resulting in a leading cause of amputations

- Premature blindness and other eye problems

- Heart disease

- Stroke

- Skin problems

- Kidney failure

Patients can reduce their risk of these advanced complications of diabetes, and prevent the onset of the disease itself. As pointed out by numerous medical research articles, a few of which are highlighted here, this is not a sort of "miracle cure." It is based on solid science, and I have observed this kind of reversal in clients that I have worked with.

Effect of Weight Loss With Lifestyle Intervention on Risk of Diabetes[27]

Researchers here were interested in finding out if diabetes prevention strategies, specifically weight loss, nutrition and physical exercise had any positive effect on the reduction of incidences of type 2 diabetes. Over 1,000 participants were followed for over three years, with the authors coming to several conclusions.

Primarily, that weight loss resulted in a huge reduction of diagnoses of diabetes. Specifically, for each 2.2 pounds (or 1 kg), "there was a 16% reduction in risk, adjusted for changes in diet and activity."[28] Even those who did not meet their weight loss goals, but who met their physical activity goal, had a 44% lower diabetes incidence.

---

27 Hamman et al., "Effect of Weight Loss With Lifestyle Intervention on Risk of Diabetes."

28 Ibid.

Changes in Insulin Secretion and Insulin Sensitivity in Relation to the Glycemic Outcomes in Subjects With Impaired Glucose Tolerance in the Indian Diabetes Prevention Programme-1 (IDPP-1)[29]

This study is unique in that it included individuals with normal blood sugar levels, those with impaired blood glucose regulation or insulin resistance, and individuals already diagnosed with diabetes. Utilizing measurements of insulin production, blood glucose levels and blood insulin that were taken at the beginning of the research, and then at the end of the three year study, several positive conclusions were noted.

Primarily that the individuals who participated in interventions including diet, exercise and medication with Metformin ™, had a reduced risk of developing diabetes. Even among those participants that had documented impaired blood glucose regulation and/or diabetes, the interventions "facilitated reversal to NGT (normal glucose tolerance.)" Interestingly, the group that had additional interventions beyond medication, "had higher rates of NGT and lower rates of diabetes."

---

29 Snehalatha et al., "Changes in Insulin Secretion and Insulin Sensitivity in Relation to the Glycemic Outcomes in Subjects With Impaired Glucose Tolerance in the Indian Diabetes Prevention Programme-1 (IDPP-1)."

The researchers' conclusion was that improved insulin action and insulin sensitivity were caused by the interventions.

The impact of lifestyle modification in preventing or delaying the progression of type 2 diabetes mellitus among high-risk people in Jordan[30]

This study outlines how simple intervention can prevent or delay the progression of Type 2 Diabetes. Two high risk (for developing diabetes) groups were studied; the first group received general guidelines for managing their diabetes; basically a handout outlining information on diet and exercise. The second group participated in 12 sessions about dietary interventions, and 5 sessions for moderately intense physical activity.

At the conclusion of the study, the researchers found that the risk of developing diabetes was more than 28% less for the group who received hands-on intervention, and significant reductions in body weight, BMI, and blood glucose levels were also found.

---

30 Abujudeh et al., "The Impact of Lifestyle Modification in Preventing or Delaying the Progression of Type 2 Diabetes Mellitus Among High-risk People in Jordan."

Interestingly, the researchers also measured self-esteem and self-efficacy in the participants before any interventions were made. Not surprisingly, subjects who had demonstrated higher self-esteem and efficacy achieved better results, especially weight loss, than their counterparts who had scored lower on the self-esteem and efficacy scales.

Category 3: The Importance of Counseling and Coaching

Several of the above research articles point to this effect, but it's important to examine this concept more closely.

Too often people "know" what they need to do, but can't do it by themselves. They need a hand; someone who is knowledgeable and who can take them through the ups and downs of this healing process. It is not that the person is incapable of making these changes, it's just that, by working with an individual who has had special training or education related to the reversal of diabetes, the client will exhibit a much higher success rate.

Why is this? Several theories abound. One is that we all need to be held accountable, and by reporting to our health instructor, we are doing just that. Just like the piano teacher who expects us to have practiced our scales, and so we practice knowing that we will be "judged" in that aspect, we tend to "stick to the program"

a bit better than we would if were trying to learn the
piano by ourselves.

Most of us tackle our health in a piece-meal approach.
What I mean by this is that we read about how an herb,
mineral or vitamin is good for "this" or "that." You
might have heard, for example, that chromium is helpful
for blood sugar regulation. Maybe you know that whole
grains are much better for you than refined grains.
Perhaps you read on the internet that fenugreek has been
used in India to treat diabetes for centuries. In short, the
"a little of this, a sprinkle of that," approach does little, if
anything, to address the underlying cause of the disease;
insulin resistance.

A client who takes a more comprehensive approach, led
by an experienced and educated practitioner who
specializes in helping individuals reverse chronic diseases
through natural means, has a much higher chance of
success.

*Lifestyle Counseling in Routine Care and Long-Term
Glucose, Blood Pressure, and Cholesterol Control in
Patients With Diabetes*[31]

---

31 Morrison, Shubina, and Turchin, "Lifestyle Counseling in
Routine Care and Long-Term Glucose, Blood Pressure, and
Cholesterol Control in Patients With Diabetes."

This large-scale study (looking at over 30,000 patients with diabetes), examined the effect of counseling that was more frequent (once or more each month), versus follow-up appointments with a physicians at less than once every 6-months.

What the researchers found was a huge gap in how long it took patients to reach target health markers, like A1C, blood pressure, and LDL cholesterol. On the following page, you can see a table that summarizes the results of this large-scale study.

Health Markers Goals	Time to reach goals with intensive counseling	Time to reach goals with little or no counseling
A1C < 7.0%	3.5 months	22.7 months
Blood pressure <130/85	3.7 weeks	5.6 months
LDL cholesterol <100	3.5 months	24.7 months

The results are inarguable; lifestyle coaching when attempting to reverse diabetes is absolutely critical if you would like to see results in lowered A1C and cholesterol in under two years! Again, this is not to imply that you can't do it by yourself....you can. However, your chances for success increase drastically if you employ the skills of a trusted healthcare practitioner.

Only 36% of men at-risk, and 52% of women at-risk, in one study, felt that they needed to attend an intensive lifestyle management course, however.[32] The results of the study above might persuade the remaining 67% of men and 48% of women otherwise.

---

32 Salmela et al., "Perceiving Need for Lifestyle Counseling."

Why try to go it alone? Let's be honest; we all need a gentle "nudge" once in a while, and we all benefit from a comprehensive vs. piece-meal approach to something as important as our health and quality of life. Invest in yourself by working with a trained and experienced professional if you are attempting to reverse your diabetes.

> "Lifestyle counseling in the primary care setting is strongly associated with faster achievement of A1C, blood pressure, and LDL cholesterol control. These results confirm that the findings of controlled clinical trials are applicable to the routine care setting and provide evidence to support current treatment guidelines."
>
> Morrison, etal

THE MYTH OF "MANAGING" DIABETES

*Every human being is the author
of his own health or disease.*

Buddha

"My doctor says I'm managing my blood sugars well," says Clyde. "Are you taking medications to manage your diabetes?" I ask. "Well, yes...don't you have to?"

One way to look at the taking of medications to "manage" diabetes is to remember this...when you are taking medications to control your blood sugars, you are giving up control of your blood sugars. In other words, you are asking the medication to do something that your body is probably capable of doing, and the root cause, insulin resistance, of the diabetes is not being addressed fully. Medications, in general, do not heal the body; they are designed to either suppress or stimulate.

With that suppression/stimulation model in mind, let's look at some of the typical medications prescribed for managing type 2 diabetes.

"Managing" type 2 diabetes with Drugs; a recipe for disaster

The typical western medicine approach to "managing" diabetes is by using pharmaceuticals, with some diet recommendations, and basic exercise suggestions. I have yet to meet a patient who has been diagnosed with either Metabolic Syndrome, pre-diabetes, or type 2 diabetes, who has been told by their primary care physician that all of these so-called conditions are reversible. As a result, the patient typically is prescribed one or more medications meant to "manage" their blood-sugar levels artificially.

As in the example of "Clyde" above, if medications are being used to control your blood sugar levels, then you are not really controlling your blood sugar; the levels of glucose in your body are being artificially, and forcefully (these medications can be very hard on your pancreas, liver and kidneys) controlled. If you are taking any of the following medications, and you want to reduce your dependency on those medications, you MUST work very closely with your physician and your natural health practitioner. It is important to work with someone who will put together a comprehensive program for you to help you help your body re-learn how to regulate sugar levels naturally; a piece-meal approach never works, and can do harm, even when you are instituting natural blood sugar supports.

The problem with every pharmaceutical, and I am including natural pharmaceuticals in this statement as well, is that they all fail to address the underlying biochemical and physiological dysfunctions that have resulted in the disease, and they all do not address long-term blood sugar control. It doesn't matter to me if a patient is taking Metformin ™ or gulping down natural chromium to help "manage" their blood sugar levels because they heard that chromium can help. Neither one is addressing the root cause of the disease, and it means that the patient is not taking an active role, but instead is taking a passive role in their health. Further, these medications, especially conventional pharmaceuticals, can cause damage, as we will more closely examine later on.

The medications that are often prescribed for patients are designed to do one of three things:

1. Improve insulin secretion

2. Improve insulin sensitivity

3. Regulate glucose production in the liver

In general, there are three classifications of diabetes medications:

1. Oral hypoglycemics

2. Injectable non-insulin

3. Injectable insulin

Oral Hypoglycemics

In most cases of recently diagnosed diabetic patients, the first course of medication is the family of oral hypoglycemics. These medications are typically prescribed when the following patient criteria are met:

- Diagnosis of the disease at 40 years of age or older

- The patient is obese or a normal weight

- The disease has been diagnosed for a duration of less than 5 years

- There is an absence of ketoacidosis

- Fasting blood sugar levels that are less than 200

- Insulin requirements that are less than 40 units per day

- The absence of kidney and/or liver dysfunctions

There are several different sub-categories within the oral hypoglycemic drug family

1. Sulfonylureas (e.g. Gliperamide, Glipizide, Glyburide) stimulate release of insulin from the pancreas and increase insulin sensitivity. The major problem with this family of oral hypoglycemics is that the already overworked pancreas is now being further stimulated. This can result in the eventual "burn-out" of the pancreas, weakening the beta cells where they will no longer produce sufficient quantities of insulin, rendering the diabetic patient insulin dependent. This family can also contribute further to the patient's hyperinsulinemia, causing damage to other organs and systems of the body.

2. Biguanides (e.g. Metformin) work in the liver, suppressing the metabolism of glucose and its release into the blood stream. Of the oral hypoglycemics, this family does the least amount of damage as there is a much lower risk of hyperinsulinemia, However, these medications still are not addressing the root cause of the disease; insulin resistance. And, if the insulin

resistance is not comprehensively treated, the disease will continue to progress, eventually resulting in a much reduced quality of life for the diabetic patient.

3. Thiazolidinediones are less common, and work within the muscle tissue.

4. Glucosidase inhibitors, again, are less common, and work within the small intestine.

5. Meglitinide stimulates the release of insulin from the pancreas.

In addition to what is mentioned above, all oral hypoglycemics come with their own share of published side effects and adverse effects.

Sulfonylureas, one of the most commonly prescribed categories of oral hypoglycemics, can cause severe adverse effects, especially to the hematologic (blood, blood vessels, and blood forming organs like the spleen and bone marrow) system; specifically, anemias, and low platelet counts.[33] There are other adverse effects that affect the gastrointestinal systems, heart rates, and hyper-sensitivity to the sun.[34]

---

33 Lilley, Harrington, and Snyder, *Pharmacology and the nursing process.*

34 Ibid.

Metformin ™ primarily effects the gastrointestinal tract, and can result in abdominal bloating, nausea, cramping, and diarrhea.[35] Though usually self-limiting, these side-effects can become quite debilitating to those who experience it. Less common, but more serious, is that Metformin ™ and similar biguanide medications can result in a reduction in B12 levels; a necessary nutrient.[36]

Injectable Non-Insulin

A recent development in the medicinal "control" of blood sugar levels are the injectable non-insulin diabetes medicines. Typically these medications are taken using a pre-filled pen, and taken either once a day, twice daily, or before meals, depending on the specific type of medication prescribed. Some examples of non-insulin injectable medications include Exenatide and Symlin.

Non-insulin injectables typically work in one or more of the following ways:

- Stimulating the beta cells in the pancreas to release more insulin when blood sugar is high. We've already discussed the problem with this kind of medication; it simply adds to the problem of insulin resistance and wears out the pancreas before its time.

---

35 Ibid.

36 "Non-Insulin Injectable Diabetes Medications."

- By suppressing the liver from releasing sugar into the bloodstream

- By slowing the movement of food through the stomach so sugar enters the blood more slowly. Again, a suppression model; better to eat food that naturally moves through the digestive system slowly; high fiber foods like leafy vegetables, legumes and beans, fibrous fruit, etc.

Side effects for injectable non-insulin medications primarily affect the gastrointestinal system, primarily via nausea and vomiting.

Injectable Insulin

Usually reserved for advanced cases of diabetes as the disease has progressed to the point that the beta cells in the pancreas are no longer producing adequate amounts of insulin, or the insulin sensitivity has progressed to the point that the cells are not getting enough glucose to function properly. The attempt here is to to flood the insulin receptors and get glucose uptake by cells.

You can probably see the problem with this scenario. Here we have cells that are insulin resistant because of a long history of hyperinsulinemia, so we are going to further flood the system with insulin to force more insulin to the already calloused receptors, furthering the damage to the insulin receptors.

There are several types of insulin available, including rapid-acting (with a rapid onset of approximately 15 minutes), short-acting (to be injected 30-60 minutes before a meal), intermediate-acting insulin, and long-acting insulin (approved for once-daily dosages at bedtime.

The Argument Against Drugs

In addition to what I've already mentioned about the ineffectiveness of conventional pharmaceuticals typically prescribed diabetes patients (especially over the long-term), these drugs have a very dark side.

As Dr. Michael Murray, a noted naturopathic physician, states, "The research is quite clear – oral medications to treat type 2 diabetes do not alter the long-term development of the disease. The drugs are quite effective in the short term, but they create a false sense of security and ultimately fail, starting a vicious circle in which they are prescribed at higher dosages or in combination with other drugs, leading to increased mortality."[37]

Metformin, for example, one of the most commonly prescribed medications for diabetes, does not work for

37 Murray, *What the drug companies won't tell you and your doctor doesn't know.*

approximately 25% of cases, and tends to lose its effectiveness over time.[38] Eventually, many patients then are prescribed one of the sulfonylureas, along with the Metformin. This class of oral hypoglycemics may cause considerable risk, especially related to heart health, and specifically to the increased rate of heart attacks.[39]

Drugs like Avandia ™ are in a newer class of oral hypoglycemics; the thiazolidinodiones. These drugs appear to be very dangerous, and the first drug introduced in this class (Rezulin) was removed from the market because of widespread deaths due to liver failure. A meta-analysis of 42 different studies with Avandia found a 43% increase in the number of heart attacks, and a 64% increased risk of dying from heart disease, compared with type 2 patients given a placebo.[40]

Drug companies are quick to point out that their products reduce diabetes symptoms, and tell their customers

38 Bolen, Feldman, and Vassy, "Systematic Review: Comparative Effectiveness and Safety of Oral Medications for Type 2 Diabetes Mellitus."

39 Mannucci et al., "All-Cause Mortality in Diabetic Patients Treated with Combinations of Sulfonylureas and Biguanides."

40 Nissen and Wolski, "Effect of Rosiglitazone on the Risk of Myocardial Infarction and Death from Cardiovascular Causes."

(doctors and consumers), for example, that Metformin reduces incidence of diabetes by 31%. Pretty good, right? Well, what the drug companies won't tell you or your doctor is that walking for 30 minutes a day, five days a week, reduces the incidence by 58%.[41]

Drug-Herb Interactions

Many individuals who are interested in integrating natural approaches with their medications will often start taking herbs, vitamins, minerals or both. Sometimes this can help, and sometimes this can be harmful. I've outlined below some precautions to take when utilizing natural pharmaceuticals along with conventional medicine.

This points, once again, to the need to take a comprehensive approach to treating and reversing your condition. Working with someone who is knowledgeable about these interactions, as well as working closely with your primary care physician (ALWAYS tell your doctor of any supplements you are taking), will help you avoid unnecessary, and sometimes dangerous, risks.

Potassium Citrate and other forms of citrate (for example calcium citrate and magnesium citrate) are often used to prevent kidney stones. This can decrease the effectiveness of many of the oral hypoglycemics in the sulfonylurea

---

41 Knowler, Barrett-Connor, and Fowler, "Reducation in the Incidence of Type 2 Diabetes with Lifestyle Intervention or Metformin."

family, such as glipizide, glyburide, tolazamide.[42] Consult with your natural health practitioner and/or physician to verify if your oral hypoglycemic is in this family.

St. John's Wort and Dong Quai are used to treat mild/moderate depression and menstrual disorders respectively. Oral hypoglycemic drugs, again in the sulfonylurea family, increase sensitivity to the sun, and so does St. John's Wort and Dong Quai.[43] Wear your sunscreen and consider supplementing with vitamin D if your blood work shows that you are deficient. (DO NOT supplement with vitamin D unless you have evidence via recent blood work that you are deficient. Vitamin D can be toxic in excess.)

A Natural Approach

What we will be covering in this book is a healing process to address the core cause of the diabetes; insulin resistance. When I work with clients who want to heal their body, and reverse their diabetes, we focus on:

- Improving insulin sensitivity

- Reversing insulin resistance

42 Harkness and Bratman, *Drug-Herb -Vitamin Interactions Bible*.

43 Ibid.

- Regulating glucose production in the liver

- Reducing post-meal high blood sugar

- Preventing complications

- Decreasing or eliminating insulin use, with physician supervision

- Eliminating the need for oral hypoglycemic drugs, with physician supervision

Disease or Symptom?

Remember that diseases are really just symptoms; signs that the body is trying to adapt normally to an abnormal situation. When you consider the development of the "disease" of type 2 diabetes, keep in mind the progression:

Step 1: Reactive Hypoglycemia

This is when the blood sugar levels are actually running a bit low. "Hypo" means "low" and glycemia, of course, refers to sugar; low blood sugar. So, at this stage of progression toward diabetes, blood sugar levels actually show on the low end; below 75, for example.

Symptoms of hypoglycemia include irritability, sweating, confusion or "brain fog," and general malaise. When things progress, and the systemic hypoglycemia episode is not resolved, more serious symptoms occur, including coma. In the most extreme state, death will occur, as your body absolutely needs glucose to function.

Step 2: Insulin resistance and Hyperinsulinemia

See "The Insulin Trap" chapter for detailed information about what is happening in this step. But, in short, and the bottom line is that glucose, the vital fuel for all of your cells, is NOT getting into your cells because the insulin receptors are insensitive to the hormone of insulin that allows the glucose to move from your blood stream into your cells. Blood sugar levels, when tested, will run above optimal levels of 75-86. Even when a person's blood sugar (or glucose) levels are within the lab reference range, or the range that the testing lab has determined to be "normal," oftentimes they are still too high, and indicate the movement toward full blown diabetes.

This insulin resistance leads to an excess of insulin in the bloodstream as well. Excess insulin causes a myriad of problems in the body (again, see "The Insulin Trap," for more details) including weight gain, the body's unwillingness to "release" stored fat, making it VERY difficult to lose weight, and a status known as hyperinsulinemia ("hyper" meaning "high," or high insulin levels). Over time, this creates an environment where the pancreas is pushing out insulin to the point where it is not really paying attention to insulin need; in other words, insulin production becomes disconnected with demand, and the pancreas, expecting the high sugar levels to continue, works overtime to produce insulin, even if blood sugar levels don't call for it. This creates a dangerous cycle where a key organ is working "rogue," and further complicating an already harmful pattern in the body.

One time a client visited with me to learn more about how she could lose weight in a healthy way. As I was reviewing her blood work, I noticed that her fasting glucose was 99. I mentioned that level was a little higher than the optimal range of 75-86, as it indicates a movement toward eventual diabetes if it is not addressed in a healthful way. It was the first time that I actually had a client express relief upon hearing this news, stating, "I'm so glad to hear you say that."

When I asked why, she stated that she had recently been to her primary care physician to review the same blood work that she and I were looking at together. She told me that she had expressed concern to her doctor about her rising blood sugar levels, which, by the way, were within the "Normal" lab reference range. She added that over the last few years, she had noticed that her fasting glucose had risen from an average of 80 to now almost 100. Her doctor stated, "Well, you don't have diabetes, yet. When you do, I can prescribe some medications to help you control your blood sugar."

I still tell this story to clients, as I think it points out several problems. First, the client had expressed interest to her physician about slowly rising glucose levels, and those concerns were basically dismissed. But, more importantly, the doctor assumed that my client would eventually progress to diabetes ("Well, you don't have diabetes, yet. When you do...), as if it were a foregone conclusion or a "natural" aspect to aging. (In fact, this statement from my client's physician is, in part, why I wrote this book; we have a mentality in our country that certain diseases are inevitable and age-related. Unfortunately, for many of us, that's true; but only because we are not taking control of the situation. This book is written to help YOU take control of YOUR health.)

But, even more disturbing in this physician's statement that, "I can prescribe medications to help you control your blood sugar." No mention of interventions that my client could take TODAY to reduce her chances of progressing to type 2 diabetes. Simple, inexpensive actions that she could take related to diet, stress management, and exercise, to totally avoid full blown diabetes.

I recommended to my client that she ask her physician to order Hemoglobin A1C; this is a measurement of glucose levels over a three-month window. One blood sample can give us an idea of how our client is managing blood sugar over a 2-3 month window. When I checked back in with my client a month later, she stated that the doctor could not order the test since it was not "medically necessary," and that her insurance would not cover it. Instead, the Chiropractic Physician in the office ordered the test for our client; total cost, less than $25.

When we got those results back, we saw an elevated A1C level; outside the lab reference range and definitely outside of the optimal range of around 4.5. The results of her fasting glucose, along with the high levels of A1C, were consistent with a pattern of insulin resistance. Fortunately, this patient, as demonstrated by her expressed concern to her physician, was ready to make the changes needed to improve her body's ability to regulate blood sugars.

"Diabetes – the First Year"

The above title came from a flyer that I saw, advertising a "Living with Diabetes" workshop series being offered in a nearby community. The class was designed, per the advertisement, to help people understand how, after a recent diagnosis of diabetes, life would be. I met with a client who had recently attended a similar workshop, and she showed me the materials and instructional booklets that were given to her.

Although an admirable attempt to educate the newly diagnosed individual, I was very disappointed in the tone of the booklets and materials, as there was no hint that, especially when first diagnosed, before the standard fare of pharmaceuticals has ravaged the pancreas and/or liver, type 2 diabetes is typically reversible.

Instead, there were paragraphs upon paragraphs either stating directly, or simply implying, that this early-death causing disease was now a permanent part of the patient's life, and that the medications would have to be taken for the rest of their lives. As we've discussed above, these medications only suppress or stimulate things in the body, and NEVER go to the root cause of the reason for the development of the disease in the first place; insulin resistance.

Below are some quotes from a variety of materials provided to the new diabetes patient. We'll discuss each one in a minute, but in the meantime, consider each passage, and write out what YOU think is wrong with the quote, based on what you've learned so far.

"There is no cure for diabetes, but it can be managed."[44]

"Living with Type 2 Diabetes." [45]

---

44 American Diabetes Association, "Where Do I Begin? Living with Type 2 Diabetes."

45 Ibid.

"No one knows what causes diabetes."[46]

"Keep in mind that taking diabetes medicines is just one of the things you need to do to meet your blood-sugar goals."[47]

Let's take each quote above, and pick it apart, if you will...

"There is no cure for diabetes, but it can be managed."

I will be making a bold, heretical statement here. While it is true that there is no cure for Type 1 Diabetes, and there is no reversal once the pancreas is beat up to the point that it is no longer producing insulin, diabetes is completely reversible for the vast majority of patients. When an individual takes absolute responsibility for his or her health by controlling blood sugar levels, using recommendations like those discussed in this book, he or she can create a situation where their diabetes has been "cured." That is, they no longer exhibit high glucose levels, high A1C levels, elevated fasting insulin levels, and no longer need medication to regulate their blood glucose levels.

If a person has completely reversed their type 2 diabetes, doesn't that constitute a "cure" of their disease? The

---

46 Nordisk, *Diabetes and You*.

47 {Citation}

medical establishment might argue that, since the disease was expressed, and even though the signs and symptoms have been erased, it doesn't mean the disease has. Keep in mind, however, that diseases and conditions are just labels to describe a physiological process in the body; a negative process where the body is trying to cope, as best as it can, with a serious imbalance. Remove the negative physiological process by taking your health in your own hands, and you have "cured" your diabetes.

Drilling, over and over and over the notion that type 2 diabetes can be "managed" sells short the power of the individual to reverse the disease; if you are told by literature from the American Diabetes Association ™ that the disease you've just been diagnosed with is incurable, what kind of hope does that leave you to feel like you can truly change this early-death sentence? In my opinion, it's terribly irresponsible for major health organizations to sell you short by implying that you don't have as much control over this disease as you might think you do. I'm not sure the motivation behind this, as the literature is fairly well established that people can, indeed, reverse their diabetes.

"Living with Diabetes"

I strongly believe that you don't have to "live with" diabetes. You can, in most cases, reverse it, and live in a state of optimal health. The term, "live with" implies that this is a disease that is yours to keep for the rest of your life. Not so, as we will discuss in this book.

If you want to live without diabetes, you probably can. By working with a diabetes counselor and following the guidelines that are set out in this book, you can shed the word "diabetic" or "diabetes" from your vocabulary. You can, instead, focus on being optimally healthy; not just being free from disease, but feeling great.

"No one knows what causes diabetes."

While this may still be true for type 1 diabetes (though several interesting and viable theories abound), the cause of type 2 diabetes has been well established for years; insulin resistance. Insulin resistance always happens before diabetes and metabolic syndrome[48], so we can safely say that the precursor to diabetes is insulin resistance. But, what causes insulin resistance? Is that known? Yes, and it has been known for more than two decades.

A landmark study out of the University of California, Los Angeles, published in 1988 in the American Journal of Clinical Nutrition, determined that there is one primary cause of insulin resistance. They looked at the following dietary and lifestyle scenarios to try and isolate the cause of insulin resistance; was it:

48 Barnard et al., "Diet-induced Insulin Resistance Precedes Other Aspects of the Metabolic Syndrome."

- High fat plus high sugar?

- High fat plus low sugar?

- Low fat plus high sugar?

- Low fat plus low sugar?

- Plus each of these diets with or without supplementary dietary fiber

- PLUS each of these diets with or without exercise

So, place your bets....what was their conclusion? The answer is that the high sugar diet, regardless of fat consumption, led to insulin resistance.[49] Further, and perhaps more surprising is that, according to the researchers:

- The effect of sugar was so powerful that no amount of exercise and no amount of dietary fiber reduces its damage

- No amount of fat restriction reduces the damages of excessive sugar

---

49 Grimditch et al., "Peripheral Insulin Sensitivity as Modified by Diet and Exercise Training."

- No amount of fat intake would cause insulin resistance, unless a high fat diet was accompanied by high sugar intake

> The effect of sugar was so powerful that no amount of exercise and no amount of dietary fiber reduces its damage.

So, to say that we don't know the cause of diabetes, I think, is extremely disrespectful to the millions of men and women (and now children) who are suffering needlessly from type 2 diabetes. Knowing the cause, as a patient with this condition, is absolutely key to understanding how the disease can be reversed......safely and naturally.

"Keep in mind that taking diabetes medicines is just one of the things you need to do to meet your blood sugar goals."

The implication with this quote is that, in order to reach your blood sugar goals, you must take medications. Of course, the booklet where this quote comes from also mentions diet and exercise, but, still, the message is clear. In order to lower your blood glucose levels, taking medications is something that you "need to do."

The truth is that, in many cases, you can naturally lower your blood sugar levels without medications. If you are currently taking medications related to blood sugar control, DO NOT stop taking them just because I am saying that you can probably do without. The healing process to help your body to be able to control blood sugars naturally takes time, and deliberate care. You MUST work with your prescribing physician closely if you undertake a program like what I describe in this book. Let your physician know that you are doing this work, and that your are hoping to reduce your dependance on the blood sugar medications. You will have to monitor your blood sugar levels carefully as you make progress, and meet your with doctor regularly in order to have him or her make any necessary adjustments to your prescriptions.

Many clients report that they are also able to reduce their dependency on related medications like those for high blood pressure and high cholesterol, for example.

"Just Diagnosed with Diabetes? Learn how to reverse it safely and naturally!"

My initial response to the workshop flyer, "Diabetes, the First Year," was to create the above workshop. I wanted people who had just been diagnosed to understand that they DON'T HAVE TO "live with" type 2 diabetes. They DON'T HAVE TO "manage" their blood sugar levels with medications. The vast majority of individuals who are diagnosed with type 2 diabetes, even if they're already injecting themselves with insulin (and further worsening the insulin resistance happening in their body), can REVERSE the progress of the disease, and, with proper TRUE management of their blood sugar levels, can effectively reverse the disease itself.

Of course, I use the term, "vast majority," to clarify that some individuals' systems are ravaged by the disease to the point of irreversibility. If the pancreas has been overworked, pumping out more and more insulin that it can no longer produce effective amounts, the disease may not be reversible. Or, if major organ systems are starting to, or have already failed (kidney failure, for example), diabetes may not be reversible. If the pancreas is no longer producing insulin, for example, the individual would die without insulin injections.

This is is not to say, however, that the program and ideas outlined in this book should be ignored; even the patient who is going in for dialysis twice a week can benefit, as these ideas will certainly help the body, and support the remaining function of the major body systems, extending quality of life, and perhaps overall life expectancy.

Your body has an amazing capacity to heal itself; I think even more than any one has allowed you to believe. You just have to trust the healing process and be willing to help your body heal by taking the best care of it as you can. What most people find when they institute these suggestions is that their primary concern is addressed, whether or not it's blood sugar regulation, digestive problems, skin issues, or any other of the myriad of symptoms that we call "diseases." But, the bonus is that they feel better; their quality of life has improved because they feel more energetic, and are doing things that they love to do, that they had given up on because of their "disease."

A radical thought? Yes, and no. Why is it radical to think that the body can heal itself and that we can, to a huge extent, control the healing process? Why is it radical to think that drugs that only suppress or stimulate can do more harm than good? Why is it radical to think that by taking control of what we eat, how we handle stress and how much we move, we can heal ourselves; emotionally, spiritually and physically?

DEBUNKING THE "IT RUNS IN MY FAMILY" MYTH

I come from a family where gravy is a beverage.

Erma Bombeck

My father has type 2 diabetes. My maternal grandmother died of complications of diabetes. My paternal grandmother weighed more than 400 lbs when she died. I have seen diabetes "running" in my family, and over two decades ago, when my father was first diagnosed, my initial thought was, "Well, I guess I'm going to get diabetes, too."

If I had a nickel for every time I've heard someone tell a similar story about their family, or chalk their disease up to "it runs in my family," I would be retired somewhere, with my feet kicked up, enjoying my vast and endless wealth.

My usual response to myself, as well as to my clients who say, "it runs in my family," is this....

> "Does the disease run in your family, or does the lifestyle run in your family?"

I am not pointing fingers at anyone; well, I am....at myself, as the "it runs in my family" statement was my first reaction to learning of my father's diabetes diagnosis. "Well, I have diabetes on both sides of my family; it's just inevitable that I will get it, eventually." But, let's peel back the layers a little bit. I don't ever ask a client to do something that I wouldn't do myself, and what I will be asking you to do later in this chapter is to examine this personal myth that you have. But, first, let me examine for you how this works in my life.

Shortly prior to my father's diagnosis of type 2 diabetes, my then-husband and I took a trip with my parents through the beautiful landscapes of Washington state and British Columbia. My mother, husband and I flew to Seattle, and met my father, who had driven from the Chicago area. This was going to be a driving trip, and drive we did, approximately 300-500 miles a day.

I learned something about my father on that trip; that if he didn't get his food in a timely manner, he got very cranky. (I've since learned this about myself, too, especially before I took control of my blood sugar regulation by implementing the recommendations that I am making in this book.) In fact, it would be safe to say that he would pitch a bit of a fit. Now, I am not judging here...back then, however, I certainly was being judgmental, for a couple of reasons. First, I was young (in my early 20s) and judgmental, and secondly, I had no idea that what my dad was experiencing was a physiological response to low blood sugar levels (reactive hypoglycemia – the first step toward type 2 diabetes) and that he basically couldn't help himself. In hindsight, of course, I realize this, but at the time it made for a stressful trip.

The other thing that I learned about both of my parents on this trip is that the travels revolved around food. There was a near obsession with where to get the next meal, when to stop, what stop had the best food, what place would have the best eats, etc. Now, food is very important, of course, but there was little attention paid to the magnificence of the landscape (the Canadian Rockies are phenomenal – if you haven't yet been, GO!), and more attention paid to the huge pancakes that we had at the diner in Calgary, Alberta.

I'd noticed this about my parents previously. Ask them about a trip that they took (and they are quite the world travelers), and they will most likely spend a lot of time telling you about their meals. Whether they're talking about the meat served on a sword in Brazil, an amazing pastry in Paris, or the grits and country smoked ham of the south eastern United States. My parents are foodies.

The good news is that they introduced us kids to a wide variety of food that I am forever grateful for. How many people do you know who more than occasionally had octopus in marinara sauce as a child, and didn't think twice. Or, did your parents ever take you to a hole-in-the-wall restaurant so that you could have turtle soup? How about a platter with a whole beef tongue set on the table? This was everyday life for me as a kid, and I am thankful that my parents pulled out all stops when it came to introducing us to different cultures via their food.

But, foodie ways have their downfall, don't they? On the one hand, you appreciate fine food. On the other hand, thinking about food all the time can be detrimental. When the activities of the day revolve around food, it can create an unhealthy relationship with food. Even clients who eat very healthfully I'll caution about this mentality; yes, we have the ultimate control over our lives when we are controlling what we're eating. However, when that control becomes obsessive and/or compulsive, we are unhealthy in a different way.

So, in my family, a near obsession with food is at the forefront. It has seeped its way into my life; I'm a foodie, too. I love reading recipe books. I subscribe to cooking magazines like Bon Appetit. I love cooking for friends and family, and revel in making things from scratch. I enjoy cooking shows. And, I love to eat...

I'm lucky, also, that my parents were exceptional at making sure that fresh fruits and veggies were always stocked in the refrigerator; I remember, too, the occasional trip to the farmer's market to stock up on local produce. Because of this, even as a child, I remember noticing when a neighbor stocked up our shared tall freezer with junk food like Ding Dongs, Twinkies, Entenmann's pastries and the like. If a bag of chips or a bottle of soda showed up at our house, I knew that my parents were having a get together or party, as those things were never in the house usually. I think it was this part of my food upbringing that helps me be as healthy as I am today; I love fresh vegetables and fruits, and I, like my parents, don't ever purchase junk food to keep in my pantry.

What else runs in my family? I've already mentioned that type 2 diabetes is prevalent, and so also is obesity. Every single member of my immediate family either currently struggles, or has struggled with having excess body fat. A few years ago, I was approximately 40 pounds heavier than I am now. My parents are both heavy. My siblings either are currently overweight, or have been overweight. We are, in short, NOT a naturally thin family. If anyone in the family is at a healthy weight, it is because we work hard at it and we have shed our excess fat. Other family members, who have passed on, were very heavy when they died; my maternal grandfather, paternal grandmother, and many great aunts and uncles. As mentioned previously, my paternal grandmother weighed over 400 pounds when she died, and my maternal grandmother died of type 2 diabetes complications (mainly heart disease).

Is there a genetic component to obesity, heart disease, type 2 diabetes, hypothyroidism, and the like? Absolutely. I am not here to deny that connection; but, a genetic predisposition does not mean a disease inevitability. It is whether or not we create the environment where that gene will express itself. So, what is really passed on between generations? Is it the genetics? Is it the lifestyle? Of course, it's both. My genetic predisposition for obesity, type 2 diabetes, and heart disease may be hard wired into my DNA, but, if I play my cards right, those conditions never have to emerge, or I can keep them in check so that, at the very least, I preserve a high quality of life.

The question to ask yourself now is, "What runs in my family?" It's relatively easy to spout off a list of conditions or diseases that "run in the family." So, let's start there. Make a list below of the conditions, and who in your family has what:

Disease/ Condition	Who has/had it?	Age of death (if applicable)

I believe that, if you have several predominant conditions or diseases that "run in the family," it just means one thing. That you can choose a different path. You can decide, today, how healthy you want to be. And, it's not just a matter of health, or even about extending life. It's about a high quality of life. Feeling healthy and vibrant again. Feeling more energy than you have in years. Getting sick less often. Symptoms of allergies being reduced. Feeling confident and fit as you burn fat and build muscle, instead of the other way around. The saying, "You have everything if you have your health," is so true here. And, you can control more about that statement than you've been led to believe.

> The saying, "You have everything if you have your health," is so true. And, you can control more about that statement than you've been led to believe. Believe...

Let's now explore what "runs in the family," when it comes to unhealthy lifestyle habits. For example, did one or more of your parents have an unhealthy relationship to food? Was there regularly junk food in your home? Did your family exercise together, or lay around watching TV? Is anyone in your family a "Type A" personality – high strung and stressed all the time? Remember, this is not a judgment of you or your family, merely an exploration to help you identify what in your background might be holding you back from achieving optimal health.

Unhealthy Habit	Who has/had it?

Identifying the poor lifestyle habits that run in your family can help you build a new path for yourself, and your own family. You can also understand more fully how and why you might fall into old patterns of unhealthy behavior, especially when you are stressed or in need of comfort. Often when we are feeling the daily tolls of life building up, building up, we fall into our old, bad habits. Think about how you might crave comfort foods (usually carbohydrate laden, greasy, or otherwise junky) when you are feeling particularly stressed or overwhelmed. By understanding your past, and how some bad habits have been with you for many, many years, can also help you understand that it will take time to reverse those automatic reactions to reach for garbage food. These are lifetime habits that will require more than a few weeks to reverse and replace with better habits.

Here are some suggestions when you find yourself reaching back into your old habits, some of which might be running in the family, still:

- When you have the temptation to indulge in a "comfort food," in times of stress, take a few deep breaths, and ask yourself what your body REALLY needs right now. In times of stress, your body needs even more healthful nourishment. Reward yourself and nurture your body, and give it what it needs to help you get through this stressful moment.

- Find healthy substitutes for snack attacks or comfort food cravings. For example, if you have a craving for a greasy burger, instead buy the best, lean burger meat you can find and make yourself a wonderful burger, served on a half-bun, or (better yet) on a green salad.

- Take a walk, instead. Find special time to clear your head, and focus on how well you are taking care of yourself – how you are taking control of your life. Your body will thank you, and you will, ultimately, heal in an emotional, physical and spiritual sense.

- Keep a journal of when you have these moments – process your emotions "out loud," to help you sort out what you're craving vs. what you really need. The popularity of blogging or journaling online via social media like facebook ™, Twitter ™ and the like, can be a fun way to share your experiences and create a support network to help you through the tough times. CAUTION: Misery loves company, and you might encounter individuals who will encourage you to "give in" to temptation; ignore them. Listen to the individuals who are supporting you on your journey toward optimal health.

Finally, I want you to consider striking the phrase, "(such and such disease) runs in my family," from your vocabulary. You are, by reading this book, and taking important steps toward health, creating a new dynamic for you and your own family. Replace the worn out phrase of inevitability with a new phrase of hope and optimism.

"Health runs in MY family."

Repeat it until you believe it – because, it is now true, isn't it?

THE INSULIN TRAP

A circle is the reflection of eternity. It has no beginning and it has no end – and if you put several circles over each other, then you get a spiral.

Maynard James Keenan

Insulin may be one of the best known hormones in the body, but one of the least understood. Throughout this book we discuss the condition of insulin resistance as the cause of diabetes, but what is the cause of insulin resistance? And, why is excess insulin so bad for you? We'll talk about that in this chapter so that you understand exactly how insulin works in your body, and the extensive damage it causes when blood sugar regulation is out of balance.

You might recall that the primary fuel for all of your 60 trillion cells is glucose. Your brain needs it to help you think clearly. Your heart and lungs need it so that you can stay alive. Your digestive system needs it so that you can properly digest and metabolize your food. Every single cell, no matter its function, utilizes glucose as a type of "gasoline" for the "engines" of the cells; mitochondria.

The balance of blood within and outside of your cells is done through the process of blood sugar regulation. Your body likes to maintain an optimal balance between the level of blood sugar in your bloodstream and the level of glucose in your cells. When this balance is disrupted in the short-term, the body has a brilliant way to bring things back into balance.

The problem comes when the balance of glucose between what is in your bloodstream, and what is in your individual cells, is chronically disrupted; that is, blood sugar dysregulation exists over the long-term. This sets your body up for insulin resistance, and ultimately type 2 diabetes if it is not addressed properly.

Excessive insulin in the bloodstream creates a domino effect of disease and destruction. Further, the excessive insulin in the system creates the perfect environment for even more excess insulin to flood the body. Hence the "Insulin Trap."

Blood Sugar Regulation 101 – Feast or Famine

You already know, by now, how important glucose is to every single cell in the body. The regulation of glucose in your body is a masterful system, designed to help you get through times of plenty and times of famine.

Trouble is, for the vast majority of Americans, we don't have periods of famine. So our amazing system of storing fat for future use when famine hits becomes a mechanism for, instead, a poor quality of life and an early death.

Insulin and Glucagon – team players

Much less known and understood than insulin is the hormone glucagon. These two partners work together to maintain healthy blood sugar levels. Basically, insulin reduces blood sugar levels, and glucagon increases blood sugar levels, depending on the needs of the body.

When you have a large meal (a feast), you are ingesting excessive carbohydrates, fats and/or proteins. It is likely that your body doesn't need all of those carbs, fats and proteins immediately, so a meal like this will trigger a couple of reactions.

First, the signal gets sent that there is an excess of glucose in the system, and insulin is released from the pancreas. The insulin helps move the glucose from the bloodstream into the cells that need the glucose to operate. Once they have had their fill, and excess blood sugar remains in the bloodstream, the insulin moves the blood sugar from the bloodstream into a storage vessel; adipose tissue, otherwise known as fat.

When the pancreas releases excessive insulin into the bloodstream, in response to excessive blood sugars, the primary message that is sent to the entire body is...STORE FAT!

Think about our paleolithic ancestors. Do you think they had large meals every day? Have you ever seen an overweight animal in the wild? Animals who hibernate eat and eat and eat so that they can store fat for their survival over the winter. But, that extra weight gain is for survival purposes, and is burned off during the long "famine" period of hibernation.

> There is a direct link between how well your body is functioning and the quality of the fuel (food) you give yourself.

The human body is designed and adapted to deal with this natural cycle of plentiful food and times of scarce resources. It's an absolutely brilliant system when implemented during acute times of "feast" and "famine." The trouble comes when we don't listen to our bodies, and disrupt how the body is designed. When the "feast" cycle becomes chronic, the body does its best to now adapt to this state, but while adapting to an abnormal situation, it creates a dis-ease state that is really just the body responding normally to an abnormal condition.

You might be asking yourself, "What do my paleolithic ancestors have to do with me? That was so long ago. Surely our bodies have evolved and adapted to modern life."

Fair question. But, when it comes down to it, genetic changes happen very, very slowly. The genes of chimpanzees and humans, for example, differ less than 1% despite the fact that it is thought the two species diverged more than five million years ago. Your genes are no different, genetically, than the genes of your ancestors of 100,000 years ago.[50] And evidence seems to indicate that humankind's genes haven't changed substantially for the past one million years.[51]

The bottom line is that our bodies have not adapted to more modern foods. Even whole grains, only introduced into our diets some 10,000 years ago, are not an ideal food for our bodies. Cow's milk causes numerous problems in over 80% of the world's population (due to lactose intolerance).[52] Certainly, we have not adapted to even more nefarious "food" items like highly processed foods, fried foods, artificial colors, preservatives and flavors. When you eat what your body has evolved to eat; whole foods like lean proteins, vegetables, nuts and

50 Sears, *The Zone*.

51 Ibid.

52 Ibid.

seeds, legumes and fruit, you feel better because you are eating according to your body's design.

The Vicious Cycle – When Wires Get Crossed

Every time you eat, you are giving your body fuel for the next four or five hours. The quality of that fuel dictates directly how your body will operate for those next few hours. There is a direct link between how well your body is functioning and the quality of the fuel (food) you give yourself.

If you are eating the proper proportions of healthy fats, lean proteins, and complex carbohydrates, you are giving your body super premium fuel. If you are eating excesses of any of the above, you are giving your body fuel that is too rich. If you are eating high quantities of processed foods chock full of artificial flavors, colors and preservatives, you are giving your body poisoned fuel. This concept is discussed in more detail later in this book (see, "The Most Powerful Drug").

When a "feast" cycle becomes the norm, and the body responds properly by storing fat, the systems of the body are functioning perfectly. It is readying itself for a time of "famine" so that the excess fat can be converted into energy. When that period of "famine" does not occur, the wires get crossed, and the body's brilliant control system starts to spin out of control, creating a vicious cycle that I call, "The Insulin Trap." The signal between the body in general, and the hormones that control healthy blood sugar levels become confused, as if the wires have crossed.

For example, let's take "Joe," a 45 year old male who is about 30 pounds overweight. His excess weight is a sign that this process has started, and his body is storing excess fat in anticipation of a possible "famine" situation. Over the last few years, however, the "feast" cycle has been in full play, and now the body has come to expect excessive blood sugar levels, so the pancreas is working overtime to produce and secrete enough insulin to keep up. At this point, however, the body is working on a kind of automatic pilot. The pancreas is not reading the signals of the body any more, so it will pump out excessive insulin even when there is not excessive blood sugar in the system. The production and secretion of insulin becomes, then, completely independent of blood sugar levels.

This is worth repeating, I think.

The pancreas' production and secretion of insulin becomes absolutely independent of the reality in the body. Whether or not blood sugar levels are high or low, the body is producing and secreting too much insulin at any given time.

This is the Insulin Trap. The body is trapped into a vicious cycle of excess insulin, causing a myriad of problems that I will discuss in just a moment. But, before we go there, you need to know that things get worse...

Insulin Resistance

Each of your 60 trillion cells needs glucose for fuel. In order to get the glucose into your cells, insulin is needed. Each of those 60 trillion cells has, on its membrane surface, insulin receptors which act as a key to open the glucose pathways in your cell membranes. Without the key of insulin to open the lock, the glucose does not get into the cell.

In a chronic state of insulin over-production and secretion, the insulin receptors of your cells become desensitized to the insulin. It's almost as if they become calloused and agitated, no longer feeling the insulin in the system, and no longer unlocking the door to allow the glucose into the cells. The example that I often use with clients is the fingertips of a guitar player. When you first learn to play the guitar, your fingertips are stressed by the strings of the guitar, and initially it can be a bit painful. Over time, though, the finger tips build a protective barrier in the form of a callous to desensitize you from the sharp strings.

The insulin receptors go through a similar response. The excess insulin in the system, now out of control, and being produced and secreted even when blood sugar levels are normal or low, agitates and aggravates the insulin receptors. These receptors, then, become less and less sensitive to the insulin in the bloodstream, and don't really "feel" or recognize the insulin in the system. This causes two problems.

1) Not enough glucose (fuel) getting into the individual cells, and
2) Excessive amounts of insulin and glucose now in the bloodstream.

We started with excess insulin causing the cells to now resist the insulin, causing excess insulin in the bloodstream, causing the cells to become even more resistant to the insulin, causing even more excessive insulin in the bloodstream, etc, etc, etc. This cascade of excess insulin and excess blood sugar levels eventually leads to the "dis-ease" of diabetes, which is really just a collection of symptoms that manifests into a destructive force within the body.

The Problem With Insulin

The kicker of all this is that the excess insulin sends the all-powerful message to the body...STORE FAT! So, even though your cells are literally starved of glucose, and you have stored fat, which can be converted into glucose, the excess insulin does not allow for easy release of that fat. Your cells, desperate for fuel, have no access to it, even if you have vast quantities of stored fuel, in the form of fat. Excess insulin is basically sending a message to the body that there is not enough food in the system and continues to store fat; the poor starving cells can not function properly, and the damage begins.

Insulin Overload and the Standard American Diet

As you already know, insulin is a hormone designed to help regulate blood sugar levels and to make sure that the cells get the fuel that they need in the form of glucose. As a hormone, insulin is part of the very complex endocrine system, which includes growth hormones, sex hormones, hormones to regulate fluid levels, and more. This finely tuned endocrine system is regulated by an equally complex feedback system, where the body tries to keep things in balance.

It is very unusual for a hormone to overload the body; unless the gland producing the organ is damaged, or the feedback mechanism is faulty, levels of hormones are rarely in excess. The exception, as you might have guessed is insulin. What differentiates insulin from virtually every other hormone in the body is that there is an easy way to increase production to the point of overload. Simply eat the Standard American Diet (SAD) that is high in refined carbohydrates and low in blood sugar regulating nutrients.

With the SAD way of eating, we have, quite literally created a recipe for diabetes, heart disease, Alzheimer's and a variety of cancers.

Insulin Overload and Diabetes

We've already discussed how type 2 diabetes ALWAYS follows insulin resistance due to insulin overload. No one goes from perfectly good blood sugar regulation to diabetic overnight. There is a long progression from reactive hypoglycemia, to insulin resistance, to full blown diabetes.[53]

---

53 G.M. Reaven, "Pathophysiology of Insulin Resistance in

Insulin overload leads to insulin resistance. Insulin resistance leads to type 2 diabetes. Type 2 diabetes, left to its own devices, leads to a lower quality of life, and an early death.

What 'causes' insulin overload? It's no mystery. The SAD (Standard American Diet) way of eating, compounded by stress (see Dr. Phyllis Cavanaugh's forward to this book), compounded by genetics (fully 75% of us are prone to this response by eating the SAD way).[54]

Insulin Overload and Heart Disease

Remember when we discussed how insulin works in the body? Each of your 60 trillion cells needs glucose to function, and insulin is what unlocks the glucose channels in the cell to allow the fuel to enter the cell.

Think about the make-up of your body; that is, the ratio of cells that are skeletal muscle mass vs. fat. Most individuals, depending, of course, on their fitness level, have anywhere from 25-35% muscle mass. Meaning that 25-35% of their total weight comprises of skeletal muscle; these are the muscles that move your body. For example, if you weigh 150 pounds, 37.5 – 52.5 pounds of that is skeletal muscle mass.

_____

Human Disease."

54 Ibid.

As you move, and burn energy, your muscles require more energy. Here, then, is the primary site where insulin and glucose interact. It makes sense that tissue that moves regularly would require more glucose than surrounding tissue which is not as active (such as hair follicles, nail follicles, major organs, etc.)

The most important muscle in your body, and one that you absolutely can not live without, is your heart. And, it is moving constantly; typically between 60-72 beats per minute. Just as your skeletal muscle cells can become insulin resistant, your heart cells can as well. This would mean that your heart is not able to burn glucose for energy as optimally as it would be able to if your blood sugars were tightly regulated.

Excess insulin is directly hazardous to the heart. Patients who receive insulin therapy have a higher risk of coronary heart disease.[55] Insulin also affects the arteries by altering the behavior of endothilial cells (which line the artery walls). Excessive LDL cholesterol, which is associated with insulin resistance, injures those cells, causing the subsequent damage to the artery walls, and ultimately the artery itself.[56]

---

55 Cleland, Petrie, and Ueda, "Insulin as a Vascular Hormone: Implications for the Pathophysiology of Cardiovascular Disease."

56 Ibid.

Insulin Overload and Alzheimer's

In addition to diabetes and heart disease, insulin overload, and the resulting insulin resistance, is widely accepted as a factor in so-called cognitive disorders that affect thinking processes, including dementia and Alzheimer's disease.[57]

Since insulin overload damages blood vessels, as mentioned above, insulin resistance and diabetes has long been considered a risk for vascular dementia – a kind of cognitive decline caused by damaged blood vessels in the brain.[58] In an article on the Mayo Clinic's main website (www.mayoclinic.com) discussing the direct link between diabetes and Alzheimer's, it's stated, "Many people with cognitive decline have brain changes that are hallmarks of both Alzheimer's disease and vascular dementia. Some researchers think that each condition helps fuel the damage caused by the other."[59]

Research continues on understanding why the link between diabetes and Alzheimer's exists. It is generally accepted, though, that the link is present, in part, due to the complex way that "type 2 diabetes affects the ability

---

57 Challem, Berkson, and Melissa Smith, *Syndrome X.*

58 "Diabetes and Alzheimer's: Insulin Resistance Increases Risk - MayoClinic.com."

59 Ibid.

of the brain and other body tissues to use sugar (glucose) and respond to insulin."[60]

Insulin Overload and Cancer

Cancer is an irreversible change in the genetic make-up of a cell. Every single living person has cancer cells, and the body's immune system is designed to identify these faulty cells and destroy them. When the immune system can not keep up with rapidly dividing cancer cells, the cancer can take hold. (See also how insulin overload affects the immune system.)

Insulin is a powerful mitogen, or a hormone that stimulates cell division (mitogenesis) and the activation of genes. Over time, excessive insulin changes the genetic behavior of cells.[61]

There is substantial evidence that type 2 diabetes increases the risk of colon, liver, pancreatic, breast and endometrial (uterine lining) cancer.[62] In the *Journal of the National Cancer Institute*, it was concluded that insulin may play a principal role in cancer growth, while control of insulin and glucose levels may slow or limit tumor growth.[63]

60 Ibid.

61 Challem, Berkson, and Melissa Smith, *Syndrome X*.

62 La Vecchia, Negri, and Franceschi, "A Case-control Study of Diabetes Mellitus and Cancer Risk."

63 Yu and Rohan, "Role of the Insulin-Like Growth Factor

Insulin Overload and Rapid Aging

As mentioned previously, the hormone insulin is a powerful mitogen, stimulating cell division. A prominent theory of aging purports that each cell is pre-programmed to divide a predetermined number of times before its descendants "die out." Since insulin overload would accelerate cell division, insulin speeds up this cellular aging process, creating biologically older cells in a younger body.[64]

Insulin, Sugar and Free Radicals

Your body needs sugar to survive. Your brain, especially, is dependent on sugar for proper functioning. The correct type of sugar, and in the correct quantities, helps your body function optimally. Every one of your 60 trillion cells relies on energy to operate, and that energy comes in the form of glucose. When glucose is burned in your cells for energy, "waste products" called free radicals are also produced.

You have certainly heard of free radicals and anti-oxidants, but how do they relate to a discussion about sugar and insulin overload?

The process of using glucose to create energy within the cells is called the Kreb's cycle. Through a number of

---

Family in Cancer Development and Progression."

64 Lev-Ran, "Mitogenic Factors Accelerate Later-age Diseases: Insulin as a Paradigm," -.

steps, the glucose is converted into energy containing compounds, namely adenosine triphosphate (ATP). Through the creation of ATP, several biochemical processes ultimately also create free radicals. Think of glucose as gasoline for your car, which gets converted into energy (ATP) for the engine of your car, which ultimately results in exhaust that is the result of that burned energy. In our example, the free radicals are that exhaust.

The problem with free radicals is that they're unstable and destructive. Your body is equipped to deal with a certain amount of free radicals through anti-oxidant activities such as those in certain vitamins like C and E. However, an overload of free radicals can cause cumulative damage to your cells and tissues. Over many years, the out of control free radicals prematurely age our bodies, making us more vulnerable to so called "age related" illnesses.

How do free radicals cause damage? Think back to basic knowledge of atoms. In the center of an atom is the nucleus, which also contains protons. Circling outside the nucleus are electrons, which are negatively charged. Free radicals, the exhaust of this energy-burning cycle, are lopsided molecules that are missing an electron in the usual pairing of electrons, which normally stabilizes the molecule. Free radicals, being short an electron, essentially "steal" electrons from other molecules; it doesn't matter which kind of molecule it is, the free radical will take from any type. If a free radical takes an electron from a DNA molecule (DNA being the material that makes up your genes), the remaining DNA molecule can mutate, resulting in cancer. Free radical damage is thought to be a major cause of aging and cancer.[65]

Several studies document how excessive glucose releases high numbers of free radicals in the body. In one study, researchers tracked how the number of free radicals increased after diabetics ate a meal, and how antioxidants decreased (anti-oxidants neutralize free radicals).[66] In another study, levels of anti-oxidant vitamins (like C and E) in diabetic as well as healthy patients sharply dropped after they were given a standard glucose tolerance test. The results showed that free radicals exploded to numbers that completely overwhelmed the patients' anti-oxidant reserves.[67]

The larger implication is that high-sugar foods generate huge amounts of free radicals, and a situation that is biologically similar to being exposed to cigarette smoke, air pollution or radiation. Unless sugar levels are balanced, and anti-oxidant reserves are replenished, the patient is destined for premature aging and preventable disease states.

Excess Sugar and the Immune System

It has been well known for decades that diabetic patients are much more prone to infections. However, it would be more accurate to say that diabetics are more prone to

---

65 Challem, Berkson, and Melissa Smith, *Syndrome X*.

66 Ibid.

67 Ibid.

certain infections, and some infections are almost exclusive to diabetic patients (foot ulcers, for one).[68] For example, diabetics are more prone to urinary tract infections and respiratory tract infections.[69]

Several functions of the immune system appear to be suppressed when blood sugar regulation is faulty, as is the case with diabetic patients. Leukocyte (a type of white blood cell) function is often depressed, as well as phagocytosis (when a white blood cell "engulfs" an invader).[70] Furthermore, there is some compelling evidence that improved blood sugar regulation improves immune function.[71]

By improving your blood sugar levels you can improve your immune system's function and avoid acute and chronic infections that can negatively impact your quality of life, and perhaps shorten your life.

Breaking Free of the Insulin Trap

The Insulin Trap, as I've previously mentioned, truly is a trap; a downward, destructive cycle that, left uncorrected, leads to a myriad of "dis-ease" and discomfort. Once the spiral starts, it's difficult to stop and, indeed, gains momentum if left to its own devices.

---

68 Joshi et al., "Infections in Patients with Diabetes Mellitus."

69 Ibid.

70 Ibid.

71 Ibid.

By reading this book, however, you are taking charge of this situation, and you CAN stop and reverse this destructive cycle. You do not have to continue down a road of illness. You can, quite literally, "walk backward" off of a path of disease, on to a path of wellness and optimal health. For too long, patients have been told that once the Insulin Trap leads to diabetes, they must now "live with" and "manage" their diabetes.

No more. You can expect more out of the rest of your life. You can immensely improve your quality of life, and extend your life expectancy. You can reverse much of the damage that has been started by the premature aging process.

You can step out of the Insulin Trap.

VITAL TESTING FOR OPTIMAL HEALTH

Knowledge is power

Do you have copies of your most recent blood work? Unless you specifically requested it from your physician and/or signed a records release document, you probably don't. Has your doctor explained the complex relationship between your blood sugars, triglycerides, insulin levels, thyroid function and stress hormone levels? Do you know what your fasting insulin levels are?

One of the first things that I like to do when working with a client is to examine their most recent blood work. Many times I'm surprised that basic information is missing, such as fasting insulin. More often than I would prefer, a client says, "My doctor says my blood work looked fine," yet when we request the lab report, there are several values that are clearly out of the lab reference range, and flagged as either too high, or too low.

It is absolutely vital that you have a complete blood panel when you start on a path of turning your health around. If you and I are working together, we both need to know where we're starting, and where we need to go. Additional testing, beyond blood work, can also be extremely important; for example, are you metabolizing fats, proteins and carbohydrates properly? How are you absorbing important minerals like zinc and calcium? How are your adrenal glands doing? Are they struggling? How is your digestive tract functioning? Is it working well, or are you at risk of decreased absorption of important nutrients?

Before I even feel comfortable making recommendations related to nutrition and diet, exercise, and stress reduction, compiling and evaluating as much information as we can about the individual client becomes a hallmark of an effective and individualized treatment plan. If during the course of our information gathering we find, for example, that your stomach is not producing enough gastric juices and enzymes, then we need to address that right away.

Vital Blood Work

Fasting glucose is what most people use to gauge their success or failure at controlling blood sugar levels. It's an important marker that is included in almost all blood panels. However, fasting glucose is terribly limited as it represents what your blood sugar levels are at the exact moment of time the needle is placed in your arm, and the blood removed for evaluation. Your blood sugar levels vary hour by hour, minute by minute. So, while an important measure, fasting blood sugar, by itself, is not very helpful to the natural health practitioner nor the patient.

Below is a list of important bio-markers that I recommend you have done with your next blood work.

If your doctor is not able to order some of them, you might want to talk with a natural health practitioner who may be able to order blood work. Medical doctors are often limited to what they can order depending on whether or not you are expecting your insurance to cover the cost of the blood work. If the insurance company doesn't think it's "medically necessary," you will have to pay out of pocket. Fortunately, for my clients, we can order blood work at a highly reduced cost as we are part of a cooperative that allows us to pass on a 50-80% discount on what a patient would typically pay out of pocket. Your natural health practitioner may be able to do the same.

- CMP-14 (Complete Metabolic Panel; this is your blood chemistry showing values related to fasting glucose, minerals, kidney function, liver function, etc.)
- CBC w/diff (Complete Blood Count; how many red blood cells, white blood cells, etc., along with a "differential" on what % of the different types of white blood cells you have in your system)

- Lipid Panel (At a minimum, you need to know your total cholesterol, LDL cholesterol, HDL cholesterol, and triglycerides. All are indicative of blood sugar regulation. We are fortunate enough to have a machine in our office that can measure these levels with just a finger prick, similar to measuring glucose levels at home.)
- Thyroid Panel (At a minimum, I like to see Thyroid Stimulating Hormone, or TSH, total T-4, your primary thyroid hormone, and total T-3, the *active* form of T-4. One measurement here without the other is akin to knowing someone's height, but not their weight, to make a judgment on the health of their thyroid. You need to know the relationship between TSH and T4, and the relationship between T4 and T3.
- Fasting Insulin (I really do not understand why doctors of diabetic patients do not order this extremely important test. As a diabetic patient, don't you want to know how your pancreas is doing? Is it still able to produce adequate levels of insulin? If your insulin levels are high, as we've discussed in The Insulin Trap chapter, serious damage to your body can occur. This is just a no-brainer to me, and I ask my clients to get this done at least twice a year.)
- Hemoglobin A1C (Also known as A1C, this extremely valuable measurement tracks, with a single sample of blood, a three-month average of blood sugars. Most doctors are comfortable with an A1C value of 6.0% or less. I prefer a value closer to 4.5%.)

- High Sensitivity C-Reactive Protein (This is a general inflammatory marker. It doesn't tell us what or where the specific inflammation is , but can be very helpful in determining baseline inflammation and tracking progress.)

Optimal vs. "Lab Reference"

How much time do you think your doctor takes to look at your blood work? Unless you are a patient on the television program, "House," (a popular program, no longer running, that played out dramatic episodes of solving bizarre medical mysteries), chances are no more than a minute or so. Physicians typically don't have time to analyze, in detail, your blood work, and only have time to glance and see which bio markers are out of the lab reference range. Even then, if things aren't *too* far out of range, your doctor may not even worry about it, nor mention it to you. In defense of the modern medical profession, doctor's really just don't have the time to do this type of detailed work.

When analyzing blood work for my clients, I don't pay much attention to reference ranges for several reasons. First, and foremost, depending on which lab the blood work is ordered from, the reference ranges often differ. For example, I have seen high-end glucose ranges of 98, 101, and 110. Which one is it? If your fasting blood glucose is 100, the first lab will report that you're glucose levels are high, the second lab will report that they are high normal, and the third will report that they are normal.

The second important reason that I don't pay much attention to lab reference ranges is that they are too wide, in my opinion. Again, looking at blood glucose levels, most labs will have a wide range of "acceptable" measures, usually between 75-101. But, if your fasting glucose is at 100, that's already a yellow flag. To put this into perspective, no one goes from perfect blood sugar regulation to diabetic overnight; it is a slow progression, taking years. Instead of looking for values that are out of range and point to an already dysfunctional system, why not look at values that are not *optimal*. With our example of blood glucose, for instance, an optimal level would be between 75-86. Anything higher or lower is hinting at blood sugar dysregulation which can be confirmed by looking at fasting insulin and A1C.

Finally, some natural health practitioners point out that lab reference "Normal" ranges have changed, and been adjusted for the worse, because of our declining health as a nation. There is some evidence of this when you consider "Ideal Weight" charts. Though I don't hold much stock in these charts, it's important to note that the "Ideal Weight" of men and women has gone up in the last 50 years as we are becoming a more and more obese nation.

Looking for Patterns

It is not enough to just glance at an individual's blood work and scan for markers that the lab has flagged "High" or "Low." More important, and which takes much more time and consideration by the practitioner, is to look for patterns. In other words, if A is high, and B is high, while C is low, that means XYZ.

Let me give you an example using thyroid markers:

- TSH or Thyroid Stimulating Hormone is Normal
- TT4 or Total T-4 is Normal
- TT3 0r Total T-3 is Low

In this case, a patient might be going to his or her doctor complaining of lethargy, fatigue, weight gain, dry, brittle hair and other similar thyroid hypofunction (low functioning) symptoms. The physician, glancing at the above values would probably conclude that everything is "fine." Sure, T3 is a little low, but TSH and TT4 are normal.

However, if TT4 is normal, and TT3 is low, this indicates that the patient may be having a difficult time converting the predominant thyroid hormone T-4, into the active form of that hormone, T-3. He or she could benefit from nutritional therapy to help that conversion process, and may very well be able to reverse his or her symptoms.

Looking for subtle patterns can make a huge difference when analyzing someone's blood work. For example, certain bio-markers can point to problems in the digestion and metabolism functions of the body (the body's ability to digest and absorb nutrients). By identifying this pattern, I can help my clients increase their metabolism of key nutrients, which, in turn, increases energy levels and reduces symptoms by getting to the root cause of the condition.

This kind of work is time-consuming; I often spend an hour or longer looking at a client's blood work, especially in relation to their personal health history, their family history, their signs and symptoms, and previous diagnoses. Although I do not diagnose clients, I can help them recognize *why* they are feeling the way they are feeling, and can often reassure them that it's not in their head; there's a physiological reason for how they feel. To a client who has been frustrated by the current medical model, this can be a huge relief. And, in my book, it is my time, very well spent.

Other Important Tests

Blood work is a powerful tool to help understand a client's health profile. Other tests can be done in the office to enrich and personalize recommendations for clients who may have other health concerns; these additional concerns can impede progress toward reversing diabetes, so it's important to consider them carefully. Chances are your physician will not be able to perform these tests, as they are in the realm of functional medicine (natural medicine) practitioners.

I utilize these tests for several reasons; first, they are inexpensive and non-invasive, and can help explain why a person is feeling poorly. As mentioned previously, that is extremely valuable information, even if the test is not diagnostic. Finally, these tests can be used as a sort of "gateway" to more advanced testing, if necessary. Most of the time, treatment recommendations can be made based on these simple tests, and more advanced and expensive tests need only be consulted if progress is not being made to the health practitioner and client's expectations.

- Functional Urinalysis (Measurement of urinary calcium levels, sediment to determine absorption of fats, proteins and carbohydrates, imbalances of gut flora and bowel toxicity, and more.)
- Adrenal markers (Urinary chloride, paradoxical pupillary reflex, postural hypotension to determine if the adrenal glands might be either stressed or "exhausted.")
- Zinc Taste Test (to measure zinc absorption)
- Oxidata Free Radical (to measure oxidative stress and the need for antioxidant therapy)
- Acidosis markers (Salivary pH challenge, respiration rate, breath hold, urinary pH, salivary pH, to determine if the client might be suffering from sub-clinical or clinical levels of metabolic acidosis or alkalosis)
- HcL Challenge (to test for hypochlorhydria, or low levels of gastric juices which would impede proper digestion and absorption)

Advanced Functional Medicine Tests

Sometimes it is necessary to dig a little deeper with a client's symptoms; peel back the layers of an onion, in a way, to get to the root cause. When the above tests don't seem to reflect what the client is concerned about, or if the recommendations for the client don't have their desired effect after 30-60 days, it makes sense to see if we can find out what we're missing. When this happens, there are a wide variety of tests that we have at our disposal as natural health practitioners. Sometimes a client can order these tests independently, but some testing companies require a prescription by a licensed health provider.

- Auto-immune tests (There are a wide variety of tests that can determine if you have an auto-immune condition that could be complicating your diabetes, and putting you at risk for additional illnesses.)
- Food sensitivities (Common allergens include wheat and gluten products, eggs, dairy, soy and yeast. If you aren't making progress in your program, despite following the nutritional and supplement recommendations, you *may* be allergic to something that you are eating, and that allergic reaction increases blood sugar levels.)
- Advanced adrenal gland function tests (Malfunctioning adrenal glands can wreak havoc on your blood sugar levels; an Adrenal Stress Index, or ASI, can be very helpful.)
- Hormone levels (Blood sugar levels and hormone levels go hand in hand. Male and female sex hormones can be measured via a simple blood test.)
- Comprehensive stool analysis (Gastrointestinal dysfunction can trump any of the above. If you have a preponderance of yeast, or Candida, a

leaky gut, inflammation, or other common maladies, these need to be corrected before you'll experience any real progress.

I mentioned earlier in this book how much I prefer utilizing research-based protocols as recommendations for my clients. The same follows with tests like the above; the client and I have to "research" the root cause of what is triggering their health complaint. Without this information, we may just be shooting in the dark, which is a waste of my client's time and money. Better to "press the pause button" at the beginning of our working together and address the probable underlying complications versus rushing into treatment recommendations that "might" help. With so many inexpensive and non-invasive tests at our disposal, it's foolish, and can be dangerous, to guess at things that we can know for certain.

Before you start any nutrition program related to diabetes reversal, work with a natural health practitioner who can get these tests done for you, and who will gladly hand over a copy of the results for you after sitting down with you to answer any of your questions, and to explain the results thoroughly and thoughtfully. You are the client, and you are the driver of the program; your practitioner is there to help you make good decisions, and to guide you through the lifestyle changes that you will be making. Don't just guess at what you need – KNOW what you need. This knowledge is incredibly powerful, and you will reap the rewards of what you learn about your body and its processes by taking the time with your practitioner from the get-go.

Insist on the basic tests, and move to the more advanced tests if you're not making the progress that you think you should. If your practitioner is not interested in these tests, or is unable to order them for you, find a new practitioner!

WHAT TO TAKE AND WHAT TO DO

Do or do not....there is no try.

Yoda

In addition to eating right and managing stress, there are some other important steps that you can take to help reverse your diabetes. It's important to note that there is not just one thing that you can do, or one thing that you can take, to reverse diabetes. There is no magic pill, no panacea, no matter what the advertisers and marketers would have you believe. But, there are certain supplements that are well-researched, and can complement your new healthy lifestyle to accelerate your progress toward reversing diabetes.

But, health isn't just about what you take. In fact, I would argue, it's not about what you <u>take</u> at all. It's about what you <u>do</u>. Achieving optimal health is not a passive activity. No one, no matter how talented and dedicated they are as a practitioner, can "fix" you. Achieving optimal health is not about having someone do something to you. The only way to feel great, and be optimally healthy, is for *you* to take control of your health, and be an active participant in making the changes that you know you need to make. Having someone to help you, guide you, coach you and cheer you on is very important as well (as we've previously discussed, this can be a vital aspect of your healing process). But the track coach doesn't run the race and win the medal; the athlete does.

> The only way to feel great, and be optimally healthy, is for *you* to take control of your health, and be an active participant in making the changes you know you need to make.

What to <u>Do</u>

A separate volume could be written on managing stress (see also Dr. Phyllis Cavanaugh's forward to learn about how stress can negatively affect blood sugar and insulin levels). Likewise, there are hundreds, if not thousands, of books about exercise programs that can also help you regulate blood sugars (exercising lowers blood sugar and insulin levels). The important message is that managing stress and exercising are just as important as eating right, and complementing your natural health program with key supplements.

Quick Stress Management Tips

The "secret" to managing stress is to understand that you can't necessarily avoid the stressors of life, at least not all of them, but you can control your response to things that stress you. One way to do that is to initiate the relaxation response, which directly opposes the stress response. Relaxation directly counters the negative effects of an extended stress response, as the table below outlines.

The Stress Response....	The relaxation response...
Shifts blood away from the digestive system toward vital organs (heart, lungs, brain)	Returns blood flow to the digestive system
Increases heart rate	Decreases heart rate
Increases blood pressure	Decreases blood pressure
Increases blood sugar levels	Decreases blood sugar levels
Increases insulin levels	Decreases insulin levels

Sometimes it's easy to "de-stress" using destructive habits like drug, alcohol or tobacco use, compulsive eating, passive activities like watching television, or consuming stimulants like coffee. Many pharmaceuticals are prescribed simply to mask the symptoms of stress, like anti-depressants, anti-anxiety medications, acid blockers, cholesterol reducers and blood pressure medications. However, all of these do not help the body, and can ultimately cause harm. Just as you might have to change some of your eating habits, you may need to re-learn stress management techniques that are *healing* and can initiate the relaxation response; even just 5-15 minutes a day of concerted relaxation can go a long way to reversing the destructive process of chronic stress.

Here are some tips to help you shift from a place of stress, to a place of relaxation and peace.

- *Breathe*: Take a few deep breaths by expanding your belly versus moving your shoulders up and down. A few moments of deep belly breathing can quickly calm you, relieving physical and emotional stress.
- *Walk*: Sometimes blowing off steam by taking a brief walk can really relieve stress.
- *Exercise*: A brief exercise session can help you shift your frame of mind. Not to mention the positive cardiovascular effects.
- *Listen to music*: Especially calming music if you need to relax, and upbeat music to feel more energized. Combine your music listening with

other relaxing activities like taking a bath, medication, or yoga.

- *Laugh*: Watch a funny movie, spend time with people who make you laugh, read a funny book.
- *Write:* Sometimes keeping a journal can help you "let go" of stress. You can also learn a lot about yourself by going back and reading previous entries, while you learn better how to deal with stress in a positive way.
- *Nap*: Recharge your batteries once in a while. Take a brief nap, or just lay down for a few minutes while focusing on your breathing, and shifting your thought patterns from negative to positive.
- *Daydream*: Don't listen to your teachers! Daydreaming is great for you. Take a little mental vacation

Move it or lose it!

Exercise is vital to reversing diabetes. It won't happen with just diet and stress management alone. Your body is designed to move versus being sedentary, and the more you honor that, the healthier you'll be, and the better you'll feel. Exercise also has a direct effect on type 2 diabetes, as it can improve insulin sensitivity and blood sugar balance and lower cholesterol levels.

As we outlined in our book, "Burn Fat, Build Muscle and Lose Weight in Five Easy Steps," there are three components of an effective exercise program:

1. Cardiovascular (Designed to increase your heart rate to a healthy level. Activities like walking, bicycling, swimming, aerobics classes, rowing machines and stair climbing)
2. Strength training (To increase muscle mass; weight lifting, yoga, physio balls, Thera-band ™)
3. Flexibility (Increasing range of motion; stretching, yoga, Pilates ™)

Before undertaking any exercise program, it is always wise to have a physical exam and physician's approval. If you have any of the following conditions, you must absolutely review your plans with your primary care physician:

- Excessive obesity that makes walking difficult
- Angina or chest pain at rest or with minimal exertion
- A recent (within the last three months) heart attack
- Severe valvular heart disease
- An irregular heartbeat
- Uncontrolled diabetes
- Blood pressure greater than 180/110, even with medication
- Acute illness
- Resting heart rate over 110 beats per minute

For more information on instituting an effective exercise program, talk to your health care provider; make sure that you don't overdue it. Start easy and gentle, and work your way up to more and more vigorous activities. For some more detailed ideas and descriptions of the three components of a diabetes reversing exercise program, the following resources might be helpful:

Burn Fat, Build Muscle and Lose Weight in Five Easy Steps, by Alisa G. Cook and Phyllis J. Cavanaugh

Ten Minute Tone-Up for Dummies, by Cyndi Targosz

The Complete Guide to Walking, by Mark Fenton

Yoga as Medicine: the Yogic Prescription for Health and Healing, by Timothy McCall, MD

These titles, and others, are available on the companion website for this book: www.stopmanagingdiabetes.com

What to take: key nutrients and herbs

Taking supplements is no substitute for taking care of yourself. None of the following nutrients, taken as a supplement, without also making necessary changes to your diet, managing your stress levels and exercising, will be enough to reverse type 2 diabetes. If that were the case, there would be no need for this book, nor for the work that I do with diabetic clients. Don't waste your money on supplements that, by themselves, are not going to make any substantial difference. You must commit fully to this process, and dedicate yourself to being an active participant in your healing journey.

Indeed, you can reverse your type 2 diabetes *without* supplements, which further reinforces the notion that the key aspects to this program are targeted nutrition and diet changes, stress management and exercise. The use of supplements to reverse diabetes accomplishes one important thing, however; that is to *accelerate* your progress. For example, one of the supplements that I often recommend for clients has been demonstrated, along with a Mediterranean style diet, to accelerate reductions in total cholesterol, triglycerides and homocysteine, an inflammatory marker, versus just the diet alone.[72]

You'll notice that I don't make specific recommendations in this book regarding dosages, etc. Similar to making nutrition recommendations, I feel strongly that the most responsible guidelines are those that are individualized to your personal health history. For example, if you are on certain medications, natural remedies can be contraindicated by either reducing the effect of your medication, or complicating side-effects that may exist for both your medication and the natural remedy. For this reason, when I meet with a client, *before* I make any specific recommendations, I review their medication list in detail, and research any potential interactions, either positive or negative, of natural pharmaceuticals that we may incorporate into the client's wellness program.

---

[72] Jones and etal, "A Mediterranean-style Low-glycemic-load Diet Improves Variables of Metabolic Syndrome in Women, and Addition of a Phytochemical-rich Medical Food Enhances Benefits on Lipoprotein Metabolism."

Below are just a few key nutrients and herbs that should be considered either dietarily or as possible supplementation. Discuss appropriate dosages with your natural health practitioner and *always* let your physician know what supplements you are taking; even if your natural health practitioner has screened for possible interactions; you can never be safe enough! (See the chapter "The Myth of Managing Diabetes," for just some of the medication and herbal interactions common with diabetes treatment.)

- **Alpha Lipoic Acid**; reduces glucose and insulin levels[73], anti-oxidant[74], nerve repair[75]. Food sources include spinach, broccoli, "free-form" in supplements
- **Vitamin C**; Anti-oxidant, lowers glucose and normalizes insulin response[76], reduces A1C[77].

---

73 Jacob and etal., "The Antioxidant Alpha-lipoic Acid Enhances Insulin-stimulated Glucose Metabolism in Insulin-resistant Rat Skeletal Muscle."

74 Jain and Lim, "Lipoic Acid Decreases Lipid Peroxidation and Protein Glycosylation and Increases $(Na(+) + K(+))$- and $Ca(++)$-ATPase Activities in High Glucose-treated Human Erythrocytes."

75 Cameron, Cotter, and Horrobin, "Effects of Alpha-lipoic Acid on Neurovascular Function in Diabetic Rats: Interaction with Essential Fatty Acids."

76 Eriksson and Kohvakka, "Magnesium and Ascorbic Acid Supplementation in Diabetes Mellitus."

77 Ibid.

Food sources include oranges, tomatoes, bell peppers.
- **Vitamin E**: Anti-oxidant, reduces toxic effects of excess glucose, offsets negative effects of elevated insulin[78] [79] Food sources include nuts, seeds and vegetable oils. Supplement ONLY with natural vitamin E (versus synthetic)
- **Chromium**: Increases insulin function[80], reverses insulin resistance[81]. Food sources include onions, tomatoes, brewer's yeast, and oysters. Supplement with chromium picolinate.
- **Zinc**: Helps pancreas produce insulin[82], increases insulin effectiveness[83]. Food sources include oysters, beans, nuts, chicken, lean red meat.

---

78 Rimm et al., "Vitamin E Consumption and the Risk of Coronary Heart Disease in Men."

79 Stampfer et al., "Vitamin E Consumption and the Risk of Coronary Disease in Women."

80 Anderson et al., "Elevated Intakes of Supplemental Chromium Improve Glucose and Insulin Variables in Individuals With Type 2 Diabetes."

81 Ibid.

82 Singh et al., "Current Zinc Intake and Risk of Diabetes and Coronary Artery Disease and Factors Associated with Insulin Resistance in Rural and Urban Populations of North India."

83 Ibid.

- **Magnesium**: Aids in glucose regulation[84], maintains insulin sensitivity[85], reverses insulin resistance[86]. Food sources include spinach and other leafy greens, beans, and nuts. Take a B complex vitamin along with any supplemental magnesium.
- **Vitamin A**: Increases insulin sensitivity[87], increases HDL cholesterol levels[88]. Food sources include carrots, sweet potatoes, spinach, beef liver. Supplemental beta-carotene is often not metabolized well by diabetics, so you may need to supplement directly with vitamin A. Supplement carefully, as vitamin A can be toxic in excess. Pregnant women, especially, should not supplement vitamin A unless under the specific instruction of a licensed medical professional.

84 Paolisso et al., "Daily Magnesium Supplements Improve Glucose Handling in Elderly Subjects."

85 Eriksson and Kohvakka, "Magnesium and Ascorbic Acid Supplementation in Diabetes Mellitus."

86 Paolisso et al., "Daily Magnesium Supplements Improve Glucose Handling in Elderly Subjects."

87 Kiefer et al., "Retinaldehyde Dehydrogenase 1 Coordinates Hepatic Gluconeogenesis and Lipid Metabolism."

88 Ibid.

- **Coenzyme Q10**: Anti-oxidant[89], reduces blood pressure[90], decreases insulin resistance[91]. Food sources include fish, organ meats, wheat germ. If an oil based supplement, take with a meal if.
- **Vitamin D**: Increases insulin sensitivity by reducing release of insulin[92]. Food sources include salmon, tuna, and fortified dairy products.
- **Milk thistle, bitter melon, fenugreek, Gymnema sylvestre, garlic**: Controlling glucose, increase insulin sensitivity, reduce metabolic syndrome signs and symptoms. [93] [94] [95] [96] [97] In general, it's best to supplement with just one of the above herbs at a time, although garlic

89 Singh et al., "Effect of Hydrosoluble Coenzyme Q10 on Blood Pressures and Insulin Resistance in Hypertensive Patients with Coronary Artery Disease."

90 Ibid.

91 Ibid.

92 Boucher, John, and Noonan, "Hypovitaminosis D Is Associated with Insulin Resistance and β Cell Dysfunction."

93 Baskaran, "Antidiabetic Effect of a Leaf Extract from Cymnema Sylvestre in Non-insulin Dependent Diabetes Mellitus Patients."

94 Jain and etal., "Can Garlic Reduce Levels of Serum Lipids? A Controlled Clinical Study."

95 Sharma, Raghuram, and Rao, "Effect of Fenugreek Seeds on Blood Glucose and Serum Lipids in Type I Diabetes."

can be added easily to the diet and is not contraindicated with any of the above herbs.

96 Srivastava and etal., "Antidiabetic and Adaptogenic Properties of Momordica Charantia Extract: An Experimental and Clinical Evaluation."

97 Velussi et al., "Long-term (12 Months) Treatment with an Anti-oxidant Drug (silymarin) Is Effective on Hyperinsulinemia, Exogenous Insulin Need and Malondialdehyde Levels in Cirrhotic Diabetic Patients."

THE MOST POWERFUL DRUG

*"Let your food by your medicine and let your medicine
be your food."*

Hippocrates

Author's note: I have taken the liberty of "plagiarizing" myself, as most of the following chapter has been taken from a previously published book, <u>Burn Fat, Build Muscle, and Lose Weight in Five Easy Steps</u>. New sections have been added, particularly the introduction and "Food as a Drug" excerpts.

I am sitting across from a new client, who has shared with me her frustrations about her fairly recent diagnosis of diabetes. She's teary, and looks me straight in the eyes when she says, "You know, I try and I try to do the right thing, and these medicines seem to help, but I just can't seem to get my glucose levels down. I'm scared."

In moments like these, I realize the gravity of the work that I do, and how gentle I have to be sometimes. These are people who are doing their best, but are lost, in a way. If I do my job correctly, I can help them feel like they are in control of their health, and empower them to make the changes they need to make.

Considering this, I pause and reply, "Susan, I know you can do this, and I'm here to help you. I know it's not easy work, but I have faith in you.'

"Why aren't the drugs working?,' she says.

"Well, they are." I state, "They are artificially lowering your blood glucose for you, and you need that right now, but those drugs don't get to the root of the problem? Do you want to know what the most powerful drug is that can help you reach your goals?'

She nods and says, "Food, right?"

Right.

Food as a Drug

Every time you eat something – every time – you are taking a drug. This drug will affect every thing about how your body works for the next 4-6 hours. Eat well, and your body operates well for 4-6 hours after that meal. Eat poorly, and your body responds in kind, for 4- 6 hours. The drug of food can be used to help you heal, or it can be used to bring you down.

When we think of food as a drug, one that either harms us or helps us, it can be a very powerful new perspective about something that most of us don't pay too much attention to. When you put it in this framework, suddenly the beautiful strength of healing foods is revealed. What you eat for lunch is the master control for how your body works for the next few hours; circulation, hormone levels, blood sugar levels, lipid (fat) metabolism, digestion, immune system. Everything.

> # No other drug is more powerful than proper nutrition.

We are always looking for the "miracle" cure for preventing and reversing terrible chronic diseases like Alzheimer's, diabetes, cancer, acid reflux, kidney and liver disease. And, the whole time, the "miracle" is, literally, right under our noses. This most powerful drug, high quality, fresh food, can heal us in a way that no drug can, no herb, no vitamin or mineral supplement, no power drink or shake. No other drug is more powerful than proper nutrition.

You are You

This chapter will explore, in detail, a nutritional outline that has been demonstrated to help people regain optimal health, and reverse the ravages of diabetes. With that said, it would be irresponsible for me to say, "Here is exactly how you need to eat...this will 'fix' you." Unless I have met with you personally, and reviewed your family health history, your personal health history, your medications and supplements, your stress profile, your degree of physical fitness, I don't know exactly what you should eat.

You are you. You are different, physiologically, from the person sitting next to you at any given time. What you need is different, depending on your current health, your emotional state, your family history...you name it. Authors who write books that basically claim, "This is how YOU should eat," are being disrespectful and irresponsible, at best, and offering possibly harmful information, at worst.

When people come to see me, I don't just hand them a sheet of paper that has a suggested menu plan. After spending more than an hour together, sometimes two, learning about what their needs are, their history, their level of stress and other factors, I customize a program menu plan for them to start. We then meet regularly, usually twice a month, to take body composition measurements to ensure that, while they are losing weight, they are burning fat and building muscle.

So, throughout this chapter you will see the phrase, "your lifestyle educator will...." This is your coach – remember, this is not a journey that can be done well alone. Recruit the help of a trusted natural health care practitioner who has studied this work, and who has helped people achieve their goal of reversing insulin resistance and diabetes. You need someone who knows exactly how many servings of vegetables vs. fruit you should be having, how many servings of lean proteins, etc.

What, When and How to Eat

This will be the longest section of this book, and that's because 95% of this program is focused on nutrition. Without a healthy diet, you are bound to fail. There is absolutely no substitute for proper nutrition, and there's no shortcut to it. Of all the steps in this program, this may be the most difficult, but you are not alone through this process.

Diet's Don't Work

Lets start with the obvious.....so-called diets don't work. You probably already knew that. Maybe you have tried several diets, or have seen your friends attempt the latest diet. And, people DO lose weight on diets, and regain that weight back, sometimes repeating the cycle over and over in a way that is labeled "yo-yo dieting." In fact, this pattern of up-and-down weight cycles can create stress on your adrenal and other endocrine glands.[98]

Fat is NOT a Four-Letter Word

Another myth to immediately dispel is that fat is bad for you. For the last two decades or so, we have been bombarded with the idea that "low fat" is healthy, and our grocery store shelves are stocked with products labeled "low fat." Yet, we are fatter than ever, with more than 65% of the American adult population overweight, and over 30% obese.[99] There are several reasons as to why the low fat food craze of the last twenty years may be contributing to our collective weight problem.

First, when fat is removed from processed foods, sugar is added in greater and greater amounts. This increased amount of sugar, especially refined sugar, leads to increased insulin secretion by the pancreas. This can lead to what is called, "The Cookie Cycle."

The excess insulin actually leads to low blood sugar, an increased hunger and cravings for high sugar foods, and

---

98 Weatherby, *Insider's Guide to the Functional Physiology of the Adrenal Glands*.

99 "Obesity and Overweight for Professionals: Data and Statistics: Adult Obesity - DNPAO - CDC."

the cycle goes on and on and on. To further frustrate you, the excess insulin that gets pumped out by the pancreas tends to increase the storage of fat....and the cruel joke that your body plays on you is that it doesn't really like to "let go" of the extra fat because the excess insulin inhibits the release of that fat, so the fat becomes hard to lose.

A second reason why low fat foods may be increasing our weight problem is that, similar to what is described above, low fat foods are not filling. So, after a low fat meal, you tend to be hungry, quite quickly, and may then tend to eat more than you would have had you had a meal with the right portion of healthy fats.

Finally, fats are low-glycemic index foods; that is, they do not spike your blood sugar rapidly like a higher glycemic index food will (starting that "Cookie Cycle" up again). The secret is consuming the right kinds of fats, and consuming fat in the proper proportion to carbohydrates and proteins. These right kinds of fats actually help your body regulate blood sugar and insulin levels, reducing your risk of many common conditions such as diabetes, heart disease, stroke, and more.

All of this leads to the basic tenets of WHAT, WHEN and HOW to eat:

1) Eat foods to help control blood sugar and insulin levels

2) Eat throughout the day – no more skipping meals

3) Eat like you mean it – conscious eating

4) Consume at least 4-5 servings of non-starchy vegetables

5) Eat limited amounts of fruits, starchy vegetables and grains

6) Don't forget the legumes and nuts/seeds

7) Eat the right types of fats

8) If you aren't a vegetarian, eat only high-quality, lean animal proteins

9) Keep salt intake low

10) Drink plenty of water

Eat foods to help control blood sugar and insulin levels

Let's start with insulin (see also "The Insulin Trap," for more information and detail on the physiological effects of excess insulin). A hormone that you'd certainly heard of prior to reading this book, insulin helps regulate your metabolism; that is how every individual cell in your body operates.

Imagine a network of over 60 trillion cells in your body. Each and every one of those cells has a metabolic process; that is, each cell requires nutrients, performs a function based on energy converted from those nutrients, and then produces waste as a result of that metabolic process. In a way, each and every one of your 60 trillion cells is like a mini-organism that needs energy, just like you, to operate optimally.

The main fuel for your cells is glucose; think of it as gasoline. The glucose enters each cell, fueling it by the cells conversion of the glucose into ATP (Adenosine triphosphate) via the function of the mitochondrium. Insulin is like the fuel pump, carrying the fuel into the cell. When the cells have the right amount of glucose, they operate fully and optimally; like a finely tuned car.

When the glucose levels are too low (hypoglycemia) or too high (hyperglycemia), the cells cannot operate in an optimal manner. In order for each of your 60 trillion cells to recognize insulin when it happens along, each cell has receptors that are specific to insulin. These insulin receptors are where the insulin attaches to the cell membrane, unlocking the glucose pathways to allow for glucose uptake by the cells. Think of insulin as the key to your locking gas cap which allows the fuel to enter the vehicle (the cell).

When blood sugar levels increase beyond what is optimal, for instance, a meal of highly processed, high-glycemic index foods, like spaghetti with red sauce, bread sticks and a glass of wine, the pancreas pumps out extra insulin to help respond to the excess sugar. Over time, with eating habits that are high-glycemic in nature, the insulin receptors of each cell become numbed, or insensitive to the insulin itself. With insensitive receptors, lowered amounts of glucose enter each cell, tiring the cell, and ultimately the larger organism. You.

It wouldn't be so bad if the worst result of this type of pattern would be fatigue. But, that's just the beginning. Long-term effects lead to weight gain, diabetes, arthritis, and heart disease[100]. Insulin resistance is thought to affect almost 40% of Americans[101]; their bodies have to produce more insulin than is healthy to push glucose into the cells for energy production. If you are overweight and feel fatigued, have difficulty losing weight, are experiencing mood swings and you've noticed a loss of muscle mass (are your triceps flabby?), you may have insulin resistance. Your program lifestyle educator will be able to put together specific recommendations specific to help you regulate your blood sugar and lower elevated insulin levels.

By the way, lowered insulin levels help your body burn fat. Remember what excess insulin does? That's right, it increases your storage of fat. Unfortunately, your body

100"CDC - 2011 National Estimates - 2011 National Diabetes Fact Sheet - Publications - Diabetes DDT."

101Ibid.

has an unlimited capacity to store fat. By lowering insulin levels, however, you can burn that excess fat, and keep it off.

Some basic guidelines for review:

1. Insulin is a hormone that helps glucose enter your cells

2. Each cell requires glucose to operate fully and optimally

3. Each cell membrane has insulin receptors to identify insulin when it is happens by

4. When the insulin receptors get bombarded by excess insulin, over time, they become numbed, or "insensitive"

5. Insensitive insulin receptors cause lowered amounts of glucose to enter the cell, and excessive insulin which increases stored fat

6. Short-term insulin resistance is marked by low energy levels, difficulty losing excessive weight, mood swings, and muscle loss

7. Long-term insulin resistance leads to chronic illnesses and conditions like obesity, heart disease, diabetes, arthritis, and an early death

8. Lowered insulin levels help burn fat and increase cell metabolism increasing energy levels, muscle mass and quality of life

So, which foods should you avoid, and which should you emphasize? It all comes down to sugar, or more accurately the food's glycemic index.

The glycemic index is a scale from 0 to 100 to measure how quickly sugar is metabolized into your bloodstream. Pure sugar is given a glycemic index of 100. Glucose, your body's essential fuel, is valued at 100. If a food has a glycemic index of 50, for example, then it is half as "sugary" as glucose or pure sugar. The lower the number, the less likely that food is to "spike" your blood sugar levels and your insulin levels. The higher the number, the more likely it is that it will cause a rapid, and unhealthy, increase in your blood sugar levels and in your insulin levels.

With literally thousands of foods at your disposal, this book can't possibly begin to include everything you will come across. Again, your lifestyle educator can put together a custom plan for you. In general, however, you want to emphasize foods with a glycemic index of 50 or below.

Here are a few examples of low to mid-glycemic index foods:[102]

Food	Glycemic Index	Food	Glycemic Index
Peas, ½ cup	48	Whole grain pasta, 1 cup	37
Kidney Beans, ½ cup	27	Lentil soup, 1 cup	44
Pumpernickel slice	41	Cauliflower	20
Oatmeal	42	Green Beans, 1 cup	20
Skim milk, 1 cup	32	Carrots, ½ cup	49
Medium orange	44	Yam, medium	51
Brown rice, 1 cup	50	Plain yogurt, ½ cup	15

102Murray, *What the drug companies won't tell you and your doctor doesn't know*.

For a comparison, below are some common processed and high glycemic index foods:[103]

Food	Glycemic Index	Food	Glycemic Index
Whole-wheat slice	69	Soft drink	68
Bagel, ½	72	Raisins, ½ cup	64
Cheerios ®, 1 cup	74	White rice, 1 cup	72
Rice Chex ®, 1 cup	89	Ice cream, 2 scoops	61
Cupcake	73	Pancake, large	67
Wheat Thins ®, 5	67	Rice pasta, 1 cup	92
Gatorade, 1 cup	78	Baked potato, medium	93

103Ibid.

The companion website to this book lists additional resources on the glycemic index:

www.stopmanagingdiabetes.com

Eat throughout the day – no more skipping meals

Are you eating like a Sumo Wrestler? Here's how these athletes eat in order to gain the weight that qualifies them for their sport; large quantities of carbohydrate-laden (high glycemic index) foods, split into two meals per day.

In order to regulate your blood sugar and insulin levels throughout the day, it is absolutely necessary to eat throughout the day, and eat in a way that will maintain healthy blood sugar and insulin levels.

You've undoubtedly heard throughout your life that breakfast is the most important meal of the day. And, there's a reason for this. When you wake up, you've been fasting; you've not eaten for anywhere between 10-12 hours, depending on when you had your evening meal or snack. You're waking up with a blood sugar shortage, and your body needs that glucose to produce energy.

You must BREAK the FAST. When you skip breakfast, it signals your body to conserve, storing fat and burning muscle to provide energy. When you eat breakfast, you actually reduce your risk of obesity and metabolic syndrome (a series of conditions that point to developing type 2 diabetes and/or heart disease) by 35-50%.[104]

Let's qualify that a bit, though. Eating a breakfast of high-glycemic index foods (donuts, sugary cereals, bagels) increases your risk of heart disease and type 2 diabetes. Make sure to select low-glycemic index foods for your breakfast. I also recommend that you eat your breakfast within an hour of waking up, and ideally within 30-45 minutes, to avoid an extended blood-sugar deficit going into your day.

Eating low-glycemic index foods throughout the day ensures steady blood sugar levels, therefore healthy insulin levels, and sustained energy. If you find yourself getting tired after a meal, instead of feeling energized, your blood sugar levels are telling you that you ate too many high-glycemic foods and/or did not include healthy fats and lean proteins at an appropriate level.

Ideally, you should eat something every two to three hours; again, picking foods that are low to medium-glycemic index foods. Work with your lifestyle educator to put together a sample meal plan; you will have a customized reference specifically for you, and for what meets your lifestyle needs.

Following is a sample meal plan for one day:

104Writing Group Members et al., "Heart Disease and Stroke Statistics—2012 Update."

Event	Menu
Wake-up, 6:00 a.m.	N/A
Breakfast, 6:45 a.m.	1 egg, 1 low sodium turkey sausage, 1 slice whole-wheat toast, decaffeinated coffee
Snack, 6:00 a.m.	1 slice, part-skim mozzarella and ½ medium apple
Lunch, 12:00 p.m.	3-4 oz chicken breast 2 cups green salad w/olive oil ½ medium apple 2 celery stalks
Snack, 3:00 p.m.	2 tbsp raw pumpkin seeds
Dinner, 6:00 p.m.	3-4 oz poached salmon ½ medium yam 1 cup green beans, steamed

Event	Menu
Snack, 8:00 p.m.	Edamame (soy beans) ½ cup
Bed time, 10 p.m.	N/A

The bottom-line message here is:

1. BREAK your FAST with a low-glycemic, properly balanced (high quality carbs, lean proteins and healthy fats) meal within 30-60 minutes of waking.

2. Skipping breakfast puts your body in a state of conservation, causing the storage of fat and the breaking down muscle for energy.

3. Skipping breakfast also puts you at higher risk for heart disease and other type 2 diabetes complications.

4. Eating a healthy, balance breakfast reduces your risk for heart disease and type 2 diabetes complications. Plus, you'll have more energy.

5. Eat low to medium-glycemic index foods throughout the day, every 2-3 hours. Again, more energy.

Eat like you mean it – conscious eating

Do you eat on the run, maybe grabbing something for breakfast or lunch, and moving while you're eating? Do you find yourself rushing through your meals to get to work on time, or get to an appointment? Do you plan your meals, or do you just get what you get, not really paying attention to what you eat? These are habits that require change, and conscious eating is focused on HOW you eat.

There are some important physiological reasons to focus on how you eat. First off, it takes about 20 minutes for your brain to get the signal from the stomach that you are full. If you rush while you're eating, you may eat much more than you would have if you slowed down a bit. When you eat more slowly, that gives the stomach time to send that all-important message that you're done.

If you consider anatomy and physiology, and examine how the gastro-intestinal (GI) tract or digestive system is built, you can understand further why HOW you eat is just as important as WHAT you eat.

At the top of the system is, of course, the mouth. This is where digestion begins as we chew and mix our food with enzymes that are in our saliva. As the food moves down the esophagus, into the stomach, additional digestion occurs by means of stomach acids, or gastric juices, that further break-down our food. The food (now called chyme), moves into the duodenum of the small intestine, where bile (digestive emulsifiers that help break down fat, like a detergent does when you wash your dishes) from the liver and gall bladder, as well as digestive enzymes from the pancreas, further digest the food.

As the food moves through the small intestine, it passes over an intricate series of villi and micro-villi, tiny hair-like structures, that increase the absorption area of your small intestine to that of the length of a football field. In the villi and micro-villi are capillaries which allow the exchange of nutrients between the small intestine and the blood stream. Our meal then continues down into the large intestine, or colon, where additional absorption takes place, water is removed, and remaining waste is sent to the rectum for excretion.

Several problems occur if you eat too quickly, or eat under stress. We've already discussed how eating quickly inhibits a timely message from the stomach to the brain to stop eating. When we rush our eating, sufficient salivary enzymes are not being mixed with our food, and we are probably not chewing our food thoroughly enough. When the food then reaches our stomach, we're at a disadvantage already, because our food has not been sufficiently processed to begin with.

What happens when we eat under stress? We've already discussed the stress response, or the flight-or-fight response. When we are under stress, either short-term or chronic, our body initiates this response in order to survive the threatening situation. We have evolved to initiate this response when we're in danger; either imagined or real; our body redirects some of its activities so that we can "fight" or "run" away from the danger.

Some of the physiological changes that occur during the stress response include heightened blood pressure, increased heart rate and the redirection of blood flow from the digestive system to the arms, legs, lungs and heart so that we can respond to the danger. Think about it....you don't really need to digest that donut when you're running away from the saber tooth tiger.

As a result of the stress response, blood is shunted away from the digestive system, and the digestive system in turn operates very minimally in order to conserve resources. If, therefore, you are eating during a stressful moment in the day, or if you suffer from chronic stress, your digestive system is not operating to its full effectiveness, and you are not able to completely absorb and subsequently metabolize the food that you are eating. Even if you have an extremely healthy and well-balanced diet, if you are eating under constant stress, you are at threat of being under-nourished.

The HOW you eat, then, includes not just the speed that you are eating, nor just how long you're chewing, but it includes your state of mind when you eat. It's extremely important to slow down your mental state as well as your fork. Before eating, and if possible, during the preparation of your food, really focus on what you're eating, why you're eating it, what it will give to you in the form of life-giving vitamins and minerals, healthy fats, lean proteins, and digestive system healing fiber. Take a few deep breaths before you eat. Say a prayer in the form of grace if that's your tradition. Just notice that you're eating, and sit down to do it. Take your time; make the time during the day to eat consciously and completely; as relaxed as you can be. Avoid distractions like computers, books, newspapers; this is a vitally important time of the day, and you are nourishing your body for optimal health and healing. Treat it as such.

Even if you can't exactly find the time to eat in a semi-meditative state, it's important to do the best that you can. So avoid the rush by following these guidelines:

1) Eat sitting down

2) Chew slowly and thoroughly

3) Put your fork down in between bites

4) Sip limited amounts of water during your meal. Too much can "dilute" the digestive enzymes and stomach acids, reducing absorption of your food.

5) Put away the distractions

6) Focus on what the meal is giving you in regards to your health

7) Make the time to nourish your body and soul by eating quality food in a relaxed manner. Nothing may be more important for your health.

Consume 4-5 servings of non-starchy vegetables

There is always a lot of debate among different nutritionist camps regarding the "ideal" diet, but all nutritionists agree that vegetables are good for you. They are a very important source of vitamins and minerals, and we should be eating more than we do. According to statistics from the Centers for Disease Control, less than 30% of us are eating vegetables three or more times a day.[105]

The nutritional value of vegetables depends on the type, freshness, preparation and cooking technique used. Vegetables are a primary source of vitamin C, along with fruits, and some of the B group of vitamins can be found in vegetables, especially dark greens, peas and beans. Carrots and dark leafy green vegetables also contain carotene, a precursor to vitamin A. Vegetable oils are rich in vitamin E, an essential antioxidant. Calcium, magnesium and potassium, along with trace elements, can be found in a wide variety of vegetables.

105"Fruit and Vegetable Consumption Among Adults --- United States, 2005."

It's probably obvious that the fresher the vegetable, the richer in vitamins and minerals. Likewise, the less the vegetable is cooked, the more nutrients it has (there are a few exceptions, for example tomatoes release more lycopene, an important antioxidant, after cooking). To minimize the loss of nutrients, follow these tips:

1. Use the freshest vegetables you can find. Frozen is your next-best option. I don't generally recommend canned veggies due to generally high sodium levels, loss of nutrients, and concerns related to the dangers of the BPA (Bisphenol A) coating used in the canning industry, especially as it relates to young children.[106]

2. Avoid peeling your vegetables, as this layer and the layer just below contains the highest concentration of nutrients.

3. Eat your veggies raw, or steam on your stove-top or in your microwave for maximum retention of vitamins and minerals. Your next-best option is a quick stir fry or baking.

4. Purchase locally grown and/or organic produce. Although there is still much debate on whether or not organically produced vegetables contain more vitamins and minerals than conventionally grown produce, there can be no denying that reducing

---

106"Since You Asked - Bisphenol A (BPA)."

ingestion of toxins like pesticides and herbicides will help you optimize your health.

5. Eat from the rainbow; that is, eat a wide variety of colors when you are selecting your vegetables. Different colors represent different families of vitamins, minerals and antioxidants. So, if you mix the colors up regularly, you will get a wide variety of essential nutrients.

Eat limited amounts of fruits, starchy vegetables and grains

Fruit are the "perfect" snack, aren't they? Most fruits can be enjoyed with little preparation, maybe a quick peeling, and you're on your way. In general, Americans are better at fruit consumption than we are with our vegetables; still only about 33% eat fruit two or more times a day.[107]

However, fruit has a dark side; when people begin to eat healthier, they will often greatly increase their fruit consumption. This is wonderful in regard to getting vitamins and minerals, and for many fruit, additional fiber. The downside is the high sugar content and glycemic index of many fruits. Excessive fruit consumption can be just as damaging as insufficient fruit consumption, but I am not advising that you stop eating fruit.

---

107 "Fruit and Vegetable Consumption Among Adults --- United States, 2005."

You do need, however, to limit your fruit consumption to 2-3 servings. Even 3 servings for some individuals is too high, and your lifestyle educator should discuss how many fruit servings you should have each day. In addition, I strongly suggest that you severely limit your consumption of dried fruit, no more than 1 tbsp a day, as they contain highly concentrated sugars that can stress blood sugar and insulin levels.

Likewise, starchy or sugary vegetables like yams, carrots, beets, winter squash, and potatoes, often have a high-glycemic index. Therefore you want to limit consumption to 1-2 servings a day. Again, consult with your lifestyle educator to discuss how many starchy vegetable servings you should have each day.

The same goes for breads and grains. I am not advising that you stop eating bread or pasta. However, I do want to remind you that one of the key tenets of this program is to effectively control blood sugar and insulin levels. Moderate amounts of grains, no more than 1-2 servings a day, will help you do that; most people should only have one serving per day. Your lifestyle educator will advise you on how many grain servings you should have each day, and which types are recommended.

I think it's important to remind you that this book should be used in conjunction with a comprehensive plan that customizes your meal plan and dietary guidelines based on your current health, your health history, family history, and your personal health goals. Under the guidance of a qualified lifestyle educator, you will be able to formulate a perfect balance for you. He or she will be able to put together for you a comprehensive list of what types of fruits, starchy vegetables and grains, and in what quantity and portion size, will help you regulate your blood sugar and insulin levels.

Don't forget the nuts/seeds and legumes

Nuts are actually fruits that have a hard outer shell that encloses the meaty kernel. Seeds, on the other hand, are found in fruits and vegetables to produce a new plant. Both of these food sources are so incredibly rich in nutritious resources that they should be eaten every day.

Consuming just 1.5 ounces of nuts and seeds every day has been demonstrated, and awarded a health claim by the U.S. Food and Drug Administration, to reduce the risk of heart disease.[108] Of course, the consumption of the nuts and seeds has to be in conjunction with a healthy balanced diet, and one without excessive caloric intake.

Nuts and seeds are incredibly rich in nutrients, with many being a concentrated source of healthy fats (more on that topic later). They are also packed with vitamins and minerals like vitamin E, copper, manganese, zinc, and magnesium. Another advantage to eating nuts and seeds

[108]Thomas and Gebhardt, "Nuts and Seeds as Sources of Alpha and Gamma Tocopherols."

is that they satisfy your appetite so that you're less likely to overeat later in the day. Nuts and seeds help maintain stable blood sugar levels[109] and although they are high in calories, a little goes a long way.

Sprinkle nuts and seeds in your salads, have a small handful (no more than 2 tbsp) as a quick snack, add them on top of vegetables and fruit, fish and other seafood dishes. Have a snack of celery and almond butter. To help you from eating too many at any one sitting, purchase your nuts when they are still in the shell. That way, you have to "work" a bit to get to the meaty kernel, and you're less likely to consume too many. The general rule of thumb is no more than 1.5 ounces each day. Your lifestyle educator will recommend exactly how many servings of nuts and seeds to have each day, and can brainstorm ideas with you on how to integrate nuts and seeds into your daily diet.

Legumes are very carbohydrate dense foods, and do trigger the production and release of insulin. However, since they are also high in fiber, the release of sugars in the blood stream is slowed, and, therefore, the release of insulin is decelerated as well. Since legumes are very high in a variety of vitamins and minerals, as well as protein, legumes are an important part of a healthy diet.

109Mateljan, *The world's healthiest foods essential guide for the healthiest way of eating.*

Examples of legumes include soy beans, peas, chick peas, pinto beans, lentils, white beans, navy beans, black beans and other beans. Fortunately, legumes are extremely versatile foods and you can have them as part of an entree, sprinkled in salads, made into dips (e.g. hummus, bean dip) or used as a meat substitute.

Most clients do well by having 1 or 2 servings of legumes each day. Talk with your lifestyle educator to find out what amount would work best for you.

Eat the right types of fats

I've talked about fats already in this book, so let's review some of those key points before we get into specifics related to healthy fats.

1) Fat is not a four-letter word; healthy fats are essential to your health

2) "Low fat" products are often chock full of excessive sugars, increasing blood sugar and insulin regulation problems

3) Eating moderate amounts of healthy fats helps you feel full faster, and decreases your appetite.

4) Fats are low-glycemic index foods, so moderate intake of healthy fats can help you regulate blood sugar and insulin levels

With that said, it's important to consume around 30% of your calories as fat; but, most important is the type of fat that you eat. You want to decrease consumption of most saturated fats (an exception is coconut oil, which is a saturated fat, but very low in palmitic acid, the long-chain saturated fat most associated with increased risk of heart disease)[110] and omega-6 fats found in factory raised beef and pork, in most vegetable oils including soy, sunflower, safflower, and corn.

In turn, I recommend that you increase your intake of monounsaturated and polyunsaturated fats, like those found in nuts and seeds, olive oil and canola oil along with adequate intake of omega-3 fatty acids that are found in fish, flax seed oil, grass-fed beef and game, omega-3 enriched eggs, olives and avocados.

The highest quality olive and canola oils are cold-pressed. That is, the oil is extracted in a cold pressing process versus a hot press or via chemical extraction of the oil. In addition, extra-virgin grades of olive oil are the richest in nutrients and healthy fats, as they represent the first pressing of the fruit. Look for 100% "First Cold Press, Extra Virgin," and purchase high quality brands that you are sure, via certification, are actually the grade labeled. Organic oil is even better as you would then avoid consumption of dangerous pesticides and herbicides that are used in the production of fruits and vegetables.

110Ibid.

What I call "fake fats" are the absolute worst. I would much rather have you consume very; limited amounts of saturated fats instead of the "fake fats.". These are found in the form of trans-fatty acids, like those in tub margarine, margarine/butter mixes, some oils used to deep fry foods, and also in other processed foods like cookies, cakes and shortenings. These types of fake fats are derived from partially hydrogenated vegetable oils, and their manufacture came out of the low-fat craze that first hit our society more than two decades ago. The thinking at the time was to reduce saturated fats, but the substitute may be worse than the original criminal.

Trans fatty acids were thought to minimally affect healthy blood lipid levels, even as recently as the 1990s.[111] However, more recent research has concluded that trans fatty acids have a pronounced negative affect on blood lipid levels, raising LDL cholesterol levels above their recommended ratio.[112] To further complicate the situation, trans fatty acids are also shown to lower HDL cholesterol levels, putting them below their recommended ratio.[113] Saturated fats do not share this trait with trans fatty acids.[114]

111"Trans Fatty Acids and Heart Disease > Publications > ACSH."
112Ibid.

113Ibid.
114Ibid.

Some tips for eating the right types of fats, in review, include:

1. Ensure that your fat consumption is approximately 30% of your total caloric intake per day.

2. Decrease your consumption of saturated fats

3. Increase consumption of monounsaturated and polyunsaturated fats, and omega-3 fatty acids

4. Purchase and use "First Cold Pressed, Extra Virgin Olive Oil," preferably organic

5. Avoid "fake fats" like margarine and other trans fatty acids

Your lifestyle educator will be able provide a list of specific types and amounts of healthy fats customized to your health goals. Some clients are "shy" about these fats, and avoid eating fats, even after being educated on how important healthy fats are for overall health. I think this is because we've been trained for decades to believe that lowering our fat intake is vital to our health. But, let's dig just a little deeper to help you understand, in addition to the previously mentioned benefits of healthy fats, just how essential these healthy oils are for your overall health.

As I've mentioned in previous sections of this book, your body is made up of approximately 60 trillion individual cells. Every single one of those cells, without exception, has a membrane, or outer covering. Think of it as the skin of the cell; and this skin holds in all the many individual components of the cell and the protects the cell from outside threats.

The cell membrane is made up of lipids (phospholipids, glycolipids and cholesterol), proteins and water. The lipid layer is predominant in the makeup of the cell membrane. Your body does not produce the fatty acids needed for this makeup; when you hear the term "essential," as in an "essential nutrient," or "essential fatty acids," it means that you must consume the item in order to retain healthy levels in your body. If you are not consuming enough essential fatty acids, not only does your chance of heart disease increase, you are not offering enough lipids for the cell membranes of every one of your 60 trillion cells to operate optimally. This can cause further damage down the road, including oxidative stress and cancer.[115]

If you aren't a vegetarian, eat only high-quality, lean animal proteins

If you are a vegetarian, your lifestyle educator can help you create a meal plan to ensure that you are getting

---

115Murray, *What the drug companies won't tell you and your doctor doesn't know.*

enough high quality proteins and amino acids in your daily diet. There is some evidence that certain individuals benefit from a vegetarian diet, but, in general I don't recommend adopting a vegetarian diet without first working with an experienced nutritionist or dietician and a licensed health practitioner. Without that type of guidance, you may fall short in several key nutrients. For example, vitamin B12 is only found in animal proteins; so, unless you are eating vegetarian sources of proteins like eggs, cheese and dairy, you are not getting an important nutrient. If you are a vegan (eating no animal products of any kind), you MUST supplement with a B complex that has sufficient levels of B12.

Protein is a key component of your muscles, skin, hair, digestive system (gut lining), and other tissues of your body. You also require protein to manufacture the enzymes of digestion, the hormones of metabolism, and for tissue repair and growth.

Protein is found in all meats and vegetables, and the best sources of protein are in the lean meats, especially fish. Not only does fish provide an excellent source of proteins, most fish are rich in high quality fats. Grass-fed beef or game are also rich in healthy fats, as well as an excellent source of protein. Protein can also be found in chicken, turkey, and other fowl, eggs, legumes, soy, nuts, beans and in dairy products like milk and cheese.

Some clients are surprised when I recommend high cholesterol sources of protein, like eggs or shrimp. Often these foods are avoided for fear that they will raise cholesterol levels, but a large body of research disputes this. For example, in a peer reviewed scientific study, researchers reviewed the effects of shrimp and eggs on cholesterol levels. For those on a shrimp diet LDL ("bad" cholesterol) levels increased 7%, however HDL ("good" cholesterol) levels increased 12%, maintaining a healthy ratio between the two cholesterols.[116] Similar results were found for eggs, although LDL levels increased 10% and 7% in HDL levels[117]; when factored in with a well balanced consumption of healthy fats, however, the egg diet did not pose any substantial threats to overall lipid balances. A bonus for the shrimp consumers; in this study, their triglycerides decreased by 14%.[118]

Most healthy sources of protein are low glycemic-index foods, and help you control and maintain healthy blood sugar balances, which helps you reduce your cravings for refined carbohydrates, and sweets. I recommend you include at least 15-20 grams of lean protein in each meal, and preferably at least one serving of fish each day.

116Mateljan, *The world's healthiest foods essential guide for the healthiest way of eating*.

117Ibid.

118Ibid.

For years we've been told to have fish several times a week, but researchers in Japan found that daily consumption of omega-3 rich fish resulted in a significant reduction in coronary heart disease compared to eating fish just a few times a week.[119]

Select fish that are environmentally sustainable. Examples include wild salmon, domestically farmed shrimp, squid/calamari, domestically farmed rainbow trout or striped bass, domestically farmed tilapia, domestic mussels, light canned tuna that is troll/pole caught, Pacific or Atlantic cod, Dungeness crab, and pollack.

Some wild fish and shellfish that we recommend you absolutely avoid because they are over fished:

- Pacific snapper (aka Pacific rock cod, rock fish, red snapper)

- Monkfish

- King Crab

- Atlantic Flounder

- Sturgeon

119Ibid.

The following fish contain high levels of mercury, and should be avoided; have these on very rare occasions:

- Swordfish

- Tilefish

- Marlin

- Shark (also over fished)

- Blue fin Tuna (also over fished)

- King Mackerel

When eating non-fish sources of protein, be sure to eat high-quality lean proteins like grass-fed beef, lean chicken (white meat), and emphasize free-range meats or wild game.

A note regarding cured or smoked meats like ham, hot dogs, bacon and jerky; this warning is especially pertinent to those meats that contain sodium nitrate or sodium nitrites; these chemicals can react with the amino acids in foods to form highly carcinogenic compounds (primarily nitrosamines).[120]

The truth of the matter is, highly processed meat is not really meat anymore; of course it will have protein, but your best bet is to choose meats that are as close to their

---

120"Nitrosamines and Cancer."

original form as possible. Processed lunch meats and hot dogs are also often very high in sodium and sometimes also contain excessive sugars, artificial colors and artificial preservatives.

Your best bet, if you need a quick meat for packing lunches, would be to purchase cuts of meat that you can quickly cook up over the weekend, and use as sandwich meat throughout the week. Like chicken breast tenders, for example. Cook up a 16 ounce quantity, and you have 4 four-ounce servings for later in the week.

If you choose to eat red meat (beef and pork – pork is definitely NOT the other white meat), limit yourself to no more than 3-4 ounces per day (think the size of a deck of cards), and choose the leanest cuts available. Avoid consuming extremely well-done, charbroiled or fat-laden meats as they have been linked with cancer, as well.[121]

In review, here is a summary related to protein consumption in a healthy, balanced diet:

1. Adopt a vegetarian diet only after consulting with an experienced nutritionist or dietician, and a licensed health practitioner

2. Vegan diets require B12 supplementation

121Murray, *What the drug companies won't tell you and your doctor doesn't know.*

3. Protein is found in all meats and vegetables, as well as nuts/seeds, legumes, and other vegetarian sources like eggs and cheese

4. Shrimp and eggs, although high in cholesterol, generally don't harm a healthy lipid balance when other healthy diet factors are instituted

5. Most healthy proteins are low-glycemic index foods

6. Consume 15-20 grams of protein with each main meal

7. Fish should be consumed daily, if possible but, if not, at least several times each week.

8. Choose environmentally sustainable fish, and those low in mercury

9. Select high-quality sources of lean protein like grass-fed beef, wild game, white meat chicken, and free-range beef

10. Processed meats aren't really meats anymore

11. If you choose to eat red meats like beef and pork, limit yourself to no more than one 3-4 oz serving per day

There are a variety of proteins, some better than others, for both the vegetarian and omnivore. Make sure that you are working with your lifestyle educator so that you get the protein you need.

Keep salt intake low

Did you know that your body only requires about 250 mg of dietary sodium each day? Yet, the RDI (Recommended Daily Intake) for sodium averages 1,500 mg.[122] Why is this? Because when the RDIs were set for sodium, it was recognized that we are, as a society, addicted to salt, and to recommend just the miniscule amount of sodium that the body actually needs was deemed impossible.

High sodium in the diet comes from prepared foods (about 45%), the cooking process (another 45%), and 5% as a condiment.[123] That leaves about 5%, of which comes naturally in fruits, vegetables, and meats.[124] Increased consumption of sodium is tied to the development of high blood pressure, heart disease, and also increases your risk of cancer.[125]

Reducing your sodium consumption is relatively simple, and after a few weeks, you will find that foods that

---

122"DRI Tables | Food and Nutrition Information Center."
123Murray, *What the drug companies won't tell you and your doctor doesn't know*.

124Ibid.
125Ibid.

formerly tasted fine to you might suddenly taste "too salty." That's a good thing.

Here are some ways to reduce sodium:

1. Read food labels carefully to determine the amounts of sodium. In fact, I recommend you track your sodium intake for at least one-week. You may be very surprised how much sodium you'll find in processed foods; most clients are when I request this of them

2. Choose low-salt or reduced sodium products whenever available. Even if you have to add salt, chances are you will not exceed what would be in the regular product to begin with.

3. Season foods with herbs, spices, lemon juice and olive oil, instead of with salt

4. Avoid canned vegetables and soups, as they are often very high in sodium (not to mention the previously stated health concerns related to canned foods' BPA coating)

5. When you're out to eat, and don't have access to food labels, avoid "high salt" preparations or ingredients like "barbecued," "broth," "marinated," "Parmesan cheese," "pickled," "smoked," and "tomato base"

6. Pretty much any prepared condiment or sauce will be high in sodium, and quite possible high in sugars. Use sparingly, or better yet, make your own.

Drink plenty of water

Water intake and fluid balance may be one of the least understood and possibly most neglected areas of health and weight management. Approximately 70% of your weight is water, and it is vital to life itself. You may be able to live without vitamin C for a week, but not without water.

Water in your body is necessary to carry vital substances and nutrients to your cells and carry waste away from your cells. Water is also necessary to moisten mucous tissue like that found in your lungs and respiratory tract and digestive system. Water helps lubricate your joints and reduces friction between your internal organs.

Because water is so crucial to health, your body tries to maintain a proper fluid level at all times. If you consume too little water, a hormone is secreted called aldosterone. This hormone tells the body to conserve water and sodium, and results in water retention, swelling, bloating and edema. If protein intake is too low, this water retention can be especially damaging. Water retention can also result whenever there is a hormonal imbalance (similar to what happens to females just before menstruation).

It seems counter intuitive, but if you are experiencing excess fluid retention due to abnormal kidney and heart functions, you should drink more water; drinking more water signals the body to slow production of aldosterone, and stimulates excretion of water and sodium. Increasing water intake, therefore, decreases water retention, bloating and added "water weight."

Another general tip is, "don't drink your calories." Drinking calories via sodas, juice cocktail mixes, juices, shakes, etc., is generally not recommended as they are often empty calories (offering little in the way of nutritive value), highly caloric, or have a high-glycemic index. Water, of course, has no calories, but you may not be aware that water-based drinks that are not sweetened, also don't have any calories.

Some examples of what I would consider "water substitutes" are:

- Decaffeinated or caffeine-free tea

- Decaffeinated coffee

- Limited amounts of seltzer water, no more than once per week

- Water with a slice of lime, lemon or other citrus squeezed in for flavor

- Limited amounts of stevia sweetened beverages – no more than 1 per week.

You may be asking, "How much water is enough?" General guidelines recommend that you drink at least one half of your body weight in ounces of water, or a water-substitute, each day. So, a 180 lb man would drink approximately 90 ounces of water each day. I think this may be asking too much, especially when you consider that you get water through the foods you eat, too.

I suggest that you find out how much water you need by conducting a harmless experiment on yourself.

Start by drinking at least two glasses of water (8 ounces each) for two days in a row. Increase to three glasses of water or water substitute per day for two days. From this point, increase by one more glass every other day until you reach what is called a "breakthrough point." You will know when you've reached this point when you experience the following:

- A sudden reduction in signs of fluid retention

- Decreased joint pain

- More energy

- Decreased weight

- Normal thirst

Here are some ideas of how to increase your water consumption:

1. Purchase a 64-ounce bottle made of stainless steel or ceramic; fill it up with water every morning and finish it by the end of the day

2. Leave notes at your desk, or on your refrigerator, in your car, or other prominent locations to remind you to drink water

3. Work with someone else, like a coworker, friend, or family member, to make sure you're both drinking enough water

4. Add lemon, orange or lime slices to add flavor to your water

Conclusion

An entire book could be written on what is discussed in just this one chapter, but I wanted to give you an idea of the "formula" for reversing insulin resistance and diabetes. Even though I can't give you the specific formula for you, without meeting with you personally, this information can be used to help you make decisions about what you eat.

It can not be overstated; food is a powerful drug that you can use to take control of your blood sugar levels, hormones, digestive system, and, in fact, every system of your body. This drug is not something that can be taken in a piece-meal approach; in other words, it's not enough to eat this or that, because you've heard it's good for this or that. Don't let yourself fall into the trap of, "I heard that _____ is good for _____." That type of approach is harmless, at best. The ONLY way to use food in the most powerful way is to use it within a comprehensive and systematic approach that is targeted toward your optimal health.

Here, again, is where an experienced natural health practitioner can guide you and coach you toward success. We know, through a large body of research, that individuals who work with a lifestyle educator, and who meet with their coach two or more times per month, have a much higher success rate, and also reach their goals in a much shorter time-frame.[126] Take advantage of this, and let someone help you achieve the kind of optimal health that will have you feeling younger, and better, than you have in years.

126Morrison, Shubina, and Turchin, "Lifestyle Counseling in Routine Care and Long-Term Glucose, Blood Pressure, and Cholesterol Control in Patients With Diabetes."

NEXT STEPS

*The horizon leans forward, offering you space
to place new steps of change.*

Maya Angelou

Welcome to your new path. The path of optimal health.
The path of becoming a former diabetic. The path of a
new family destiny; health runs in your family, now. You
are forging a brand new trail, and it will come with
immense rewards.

Building a new path is not easy work, just like carving a
walking path up the side of a mountain requires intense
labor. But, the views from that trail, as you climb up and
up, getting stronger and healthier, are amazing; and when
you look down on how far you have traveled, you will
smile as you keep climbing upward.

It has been my true pleasure and honor to introduce you
to this new path, and I am confident that the information
contained in this book will help you reach your goals.

You are just beginning your journey, and you will likely need support, so do please work with a qualified natural health practitioner who can help get through the rough times that a program like this entails. Meeting regularly, at least twice a month, will greatly increase your chances of success and immensely shorten the time needed to reach your goals. If you work with someone who can guide you through each step of the way, you can most likely reverse your diabetes in less than a year.

This book is just one aspect of the supports I have created for you. In addition to the information here, on the companion website (www.stopmanagingdiabetes.com) you will also find:

- Direct links to some of the research cited
- Links and resources for other valuable tools to take with you on your new health journey
- Wellness program options
- Stop Managing Diabetes online tools including recipes, hints and tips, and research updates
- Online classes and webinars
- And more

I wish you all the best on your travels!

In health,

Alisa

Alisa G. Cook, C.A., M.A.
Certified Traditional Naturopath
September, 2012

ABOUT THE AUTHOR

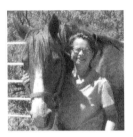

A former educator, Alisa's new role in education is helping her clients understand how their body can heal itself, given the right tools, support and time. Her clients note her sincere and respectful approach, and her willingness to take the time needed to listen to their story.

After completing coursework in anatomy and physiology, holistic protocols, holistic nutrition, holistic pathophysiology, herbalism, and more, Alisa continued her studies, under Dr. Dicken Weatherby, to include Functional Blood Work Analysis and Functional Diagnosis. She is recognized by the American Naturopathic Certification Board as a Certified Traditional Naturopath ™ (CTN).

When she is not working with people or their animals, Alisa enjoys gardening, reading, puttering around "the ranch," spending time with her numerous animals, hiking, motorcycling, traveling and cooking and having dinner with friends.

For a personal consultation, contact Alisa at 520-366-1646, or by email at gaiawellness@ymail.com

References

Abujudeh, Bashar A., Raeda F. Abu Al Rub, Ibrahim G. Al-Faouri, and Muntaha K. Gharaibeh. "The Impact of Lifestyle Modification in Preventing or Delaying the Progression of Type 2 Diabetes Mellitus Among High-risk People in Jordan." *Journal of Research in Nursing* 17, no. 1 (January 1, 2012): 32 –44.

American Diabetes Association. "Where Do I Begin? Living with Type 2 Diabetes". American Diabetes Association, n.d.

Anderson, Richard A, Nanzheng Cheng, Noella A Bryden, Marilyn M Polansky, Nanping Cheng, Jiaming Chi, and Jinguang Feng. "Elevated Intakes of Supplemental Chromium Improve Glucose and Insulin Variables in Individuals With Type 2 Diabetes." *Diabetes* 46, no. 11 (November 1, 1997): 1786–1791.

Barnard, R. James, Christian K. Roberts, Shira M. Varon, and Joshua J. Berger. "Diet-induced Insulin Resistance Precedes Other Aspects of the Metabolic Syndrome." *Journal of Applied Physiology* 84, no. 4 (April 1, 1998): 1311 –1315.

Baskaran, K. "Antidiabetic Effect of a Leaf Extract from Cymnema Sylvestre in Non-insulin Dependent Diabetes Mellitus Patients." *Journal of Ethnopharmacology* 30 (1990): 295–305.

Bolen, S., L. Feldman, and J. Vassy. "Systematic Review: Comparative Effectiveness and Safety of Oral Medications for Type 2 Diabetes Mellitus." *Annals of Internal Medicine* 147, no. 6 (2007): 386–399.

Boucher, Barbara J, W Garry John, and Kate Noonan. "Hypovitaminosis D Is Associated with Insulin Resistance and β Cell Dysfunction." *The American Journal of Clinical Nutrition* 80, no. 6 (December 1, 2004): 1666–1666.

Buse, John B., Sonia Caprio, William T. Cefalu, Antonio Ceriello, Stefano Del Prato, Silvio E. Inzucchi, Sue McLaughlin, et al. "How Do We Define Cure of Diabetes?" *Diabetes Care* 32, no. 11 (November 1, 2009): 2133 –2135.

Cameron, NE, MA Cotter, and DH Horrobin. "Effects of Alpha-lipoic Acid on Neurovascular Function in Diabetic Rats: Interaction with Essential Fatty Acids." *Diabetologia* 41 (1998): 390–399.

"CDC - 2011 National Estimates - 2011 National Diabetes Fact Sheet - Publications - Diabetes DDT", n.d. http://www.cdc.gov/diabetes/pubs/estimates11.htm#10.

Ceriello, A., N. Bortolotti, and A. Crescentini. "Antioxidant Defences Are Reduced During the Oral Glucose Tolerance Test in Normal and Noninsulin-dependent Diabetic Subjects." *European Journal of Clinical Investigation* 28 (1998): 329–333.

Challem, Jack, Burt Berkson, and Melissa Smith. *Syndrome X.* New York, NY: John Wiley & Sons, Inc., 200AD.

Cleland, S.J., J.R. Petrie, and S. Ueda. "Insulin as a Vascular Hormone: Implications for the Pathophysiology of Cardiovascular Disease." *Clinical and Experimental Pharmacology and Physiology* 25 (1998): 175–184.

"Diabetes and Alzheimer's: Insulin Resistance Increases Risk - MayoClinic.com", n.d. http://www.mayoclinic.com/health/diabetes-and-alzheimers/AZ00050.

"Diabetes Statistics - American Diabetes Association", n.d. http://www.diabetes.org/diabetes-basics/diabetes-statistics/?loc=DropDownDB-stats.

"DRI Tables | Food and Nutrition Information Center", n.d. http://fnic.nal.usda.gov/dietary-guidance/dietary-reference-intakes/dri-tables.

Eriksson, J., and A. Kohvakka. "Magnesium and Ascorbic Acid Supplementation in Diabetes Mellitus." *Annals of Nutrition and Metabolism* 39, no. 4 (1995): 217–223.

"Fruit and Vegetable Consumption Among Adults --- United States, 2005", n.d. http://www.cdc.gov/mmwr/preview/mmwrhtml/mm5610a2.htm.

G.M. Reaven. "Pathophysiology of Insulin Resistance in Human
        Disease." *Physiological Review* 75 (1995): 473–485.

"Getting Started With Diabetes - American Diabetes Association", n.d.
        http://www.diabetes.org/living-with-diabetes/recently-
        diagnosed/where-do-i-begin/getting-started-with-
        diabetes.html.

Grimditch, G K, R J Barnard, L Hendricks, and D Weitzman.
        "Peripheral Insulin Sensitivity as Modified by Diet and
        Exercise Training." *The American Journal of Clinical
        Nutrition* 48, no. 1 (July 1, 1988): 38 –43.

Hamman, Richard F., Rena R. Wing, Sharon L. Edelstein, John M.
        Lachin, George A. Bray, Linda Delahanty, Mary Hoskin, et
        al. "Effect of Weight Loss With Lifestyle Intervention on
        Risk of Diabetes." *Diabetes Care* 29, no. 9 (September
        2006): 2102 –2107.

Harkness, Richard, and Steven Bratman. *Drug-Herb -Vitamin
        Interactions Bible*. New York, NY: Prima Publishing, 2000.

Jacob, S, and etal. "The Antioxidant Alpha-lipoic Acid Enhances
        Insulin-stimulated Glucose Metabolism in Insulin-resistant
        Rat Skeletal Muscle." *Diabetes* 45 (1996): 1024–1029.

Jain, AK, and etal. "Can Garlic Reduce Levels of Serum Lipids? A
        Controlled Clinical Study." *American Journal of Medicine*
        94 (1993): 632–6356.

Jain, S.K., and G Lim. "Lipoic Acid Decreases Lipid Peroxidation and
        Protein Glycosylation and Increases (Na(+) + K(+))- and
        Ca(++)-ATPase Activities in High Glucose-treated Human
        Erythrocytes." *Free Radical Biology and Medicine* 11
        (2000): 1122–1128.

Jones, Jennifer, and etal. "A Mediterranean-style Low-glycemic-load
        Diet Improves Variables of Metabolic Syndrome in Women,
        and Addition of a Phytochemical-rich Medical Food
        Enhances Benefits on Lipoprotein Metabolism." *Journal of
        Clinical Lipidology* (n.d.).

Joshi, Nirmal, Gregory M. Caputo, Michael R. Weitekamp, and A.W.
        Karchmer. "Infections in Patients with Diabetes Mellitus." *N
        Engl J Med* 341, no. 25 (December 16, 1999): 1906–1912.

Kiefer, Florian W., Gabriela Orasanu, Shriram Nallamshetty, Jonathan D. Brown, Hong Wang, Philip Luger, Nathan R. Qi, Charles F. Burant, Gregg Duester, and Jorge Plutzky. "Retinaldehyde Dehydrogenase 1 Coordinates Hepatic Gluconeogenesis and Lipid Metabolism." *Endocrinology* 153, no. 7 (July 1, 2012): 3089–3099.

Knowler, W.C., E. Barrett-Connor, and S.E. Fowler. "Reducation in the Incidence of Type 2 Diabetes with Lifestyle Intervention or Metformin." *New* 346, no. 6 (2002): 393–403.

Larson-Meyer, D. E. "Effect of Calorie Restriction With or Without Exercise on Insulin Sensitivity, -Cell Function, Fat Cell Size, and Ectopic Lipid in Overweight Subjects." *Diabetes Care* 29, no. 6 (June 1, 2006): 1337–1344.

Lev-Ran, A. "Mitogenic Factors Accelerate Later-age Diseases: Insulin as a Paradigm." *Mechanisms of Aging and Development* 102 (1998): 95–113.

Li, Chaoyang, Earl S. Ford, Ali H. Mokdad, Ruth Jiles, and Wayne H. Giles. "Clustering of Multiple Healthy Lifestyle Habits and Health-Related Quality of Life Among U.S. Adults With Diabetes." *Diabetes Care* 30, no. 7 (July 2007): 1770 –1776.

Lilley, Linda Lane, Scott Harrington, and Julie S Snyder. *Pharmacology and the nursing process*. St. Louis, Mo.: Mosby, 2005.

Mannucci, M., M. Monami, G. Masotti, and N. Marchionni. "All-Cause Mortality in Diabetic Patients Treated with Combinations of Sulfonylureas and Biguanides." *Diabetes Metabolism* 20, no. 1 (2004): 44–47.

Mateljan, George. *The world's healthiest foods essential guide for the healthiest way of eating*. Seattle, Wash.: George Mateljan Foundation, 2006. http://www.contentreserve.com/TitleInfo.asp?ID={8BFE2665-0BB5-4A36-BBA0-C7846EA3763C}&Format=410.

Morrison, Fritha, Maria Shubina, and Alexander Turchin. "Lifestyle Counseling in Routine Care and Long-Term Glucose, Blood Pressure, and Cholesterol Control in Patients With Diabetes." *Diabetes Care* 35, no. 2 (February 1, 2012): 334 341.

Murray, Michael T. *What the drug companies won't tell you and your doctor doesn't know : the alternative treatments that may change your life-- and the prescriptions that could harm you.* New York: Atria Paperbacks, 2010.

Nissen, S.E., and K. Wolski. "Effect of Rosiglitazone on the Risk of Myocardial Infarction and Death from Cardiovascular Causes." *New England Journal of Medicine* 356, no. 24 (2007): 2457–2471.

"Nitrosamines and Cancer", n.d. http://lpi.oregonstate.edu/f-w00/nitrosamine.html/.

"Non-Insulin Injectable Diabetes Medications", n.d. http://my.clevelandclinic.org/disorders/diabetes_mellitus/hic_non-insulin_injectable_medications.aspx.

Nordisk, Novo. *Diabetes and You.* U.S.A.: Cornerstones4Care, 2011.

"Obesity and Overweight for Professionals: Data and Statistics: Adult Obesity - DNPAO - CDC", n.d. http://www.cdc.gov/obesity/data/adult.html.

Paolisso, G, S Sgambato, A Gambardella, and etal. "Daily Magnesium Supplements Improve Glucose Handling in Elderly Subjects." *American Journal of Clinical Nutrition* 55 (1992): 1161–1167.

Rimm, Eric B., Meir J. Stampfer, Alberto Ascherio, Edward Giovannucci, Graham A. Colditz, and Walter C. Willett. "Vitamin E Consumption and the Risk of Coronary Heart Disease in Men." *New England Journal of Medicine* 328, no. 20 (May 20, 1993): 1450–1456.

Salmela, Sanna M., Kati A. Vähäsarja, Jari J. Villberg, Mauno J. Vanhala, Timo E. Saaristo, Jaana Lindström, Heikki H. Oksa, et al. "Perceiving Need for Lifestyle Counseling." *Diabetes Care* 35, no. 2 (February 1, 2012): 239 –241.

Sears, Barry. *The Zone.* New York, NY: HarperCollins, 1995.

Sharma, RD, TC Raghuram, and NS Rao. "Effect of Fenugreek Seeds on Blood Glucose and Serum Lipids in Type I Diabetes." *European Journal of Clinical Nutrition* 44 (1990): 301–306.

"Since You Asked - Bisphenol A (BPA)", n.d. http://www.niehs.nih.gov/news/sya/sya-bpa/.

Singh, Ram B., Mohammad A. Niaz, Shanti S. Rastogi, Sarita Bajaj, Zhang Gaoli, and Zhu Shoumin. "Current Zinc Intake and Risk of Diabetes and Coronary Artery Disease and Factors Associated with Insulin Resistance in Rural and Urban Populations of North India." *Journal of the American College of Nutrition* 17, no. 6 (December 1, 1998): 564–570.

Singh, RB, MA Niaz, SS Rastogi, PK Shukla, and AS Thakur. "Effect of Hydrosoluble Coenzyme Q10 on Blood Pressures and Insulin Resistance in Hypertensive Patients with Coronary Artery Disease." *Journal of Human Hypertension* 13, no. 3 (March 1999): 203–208.

Snehalatha, Chamukuttan, Simon Mary, Sundaram Selvam, Cholaiyil Kizhakathil Sathish Kumar, Samith Babu Ananth Shetty, Arun Nanditha, and Ambady Ramachandran. "Changes in Insulin Secretion and Insulin Sensitivity in Relation to the Glycemic Outcomes in Subjects With Impaired Glucose Tolerance in the Indian Diabetes Prevention Programme-1 (IDPP-1)." *Diabetes Care* 32, no. 10 (October 1, 2009): 1796–1801.

Srivastava, Y, and etal. "Antidiabetic and Adaptogenic Properties of Momordica Charantia Extract: An Experimental and Clinical Evaluation." *Phytotherapy Research* 7 (1993): 285–289.

Stampfer, Meir J., Charles H. Hennekens, JoAnn E. Manson, Graham A. Colditz, Bernard Rosner, and Walter C. Willett. "Vitamin E Consumption and the Risk of Coronary Disease in Women." *New England Journal of Medicine* 328, no. 20 (May 20, 1993): 1444–1449.

"Symptoms - American Diabetes Association", n.d. http://www.diabetes.org/diabetes-basics/symptoms/?loc=DropDownDB-symptoms&utm_expid=54551592-7&utm_referrer=http%3A%2F%2Fwww.diabetes.org%2F.

Thomas, Robin, and S.E. Gebhardt. "Nuts and Seeds as Sources of Alpha and Gamma Tocopherols". USDA-ARS Nutrient Data Laboratory, 2010.

Toobert, Deborah J., Russell E. Glasgow, Lisa A. Strycker, Manuel Barrera, Janice L. Radcliffe, Rosemary C. Wander, and John D. Bagdade. "Biologic and Quality-of-Life Outcomes From the Mediterranean Lifestyle Program." *Diabetes Care* 26, no. 8 (2003): 2288 –2293.

Torjesen, P. A., K. I. Birkeland, S. A. Anderssen, I. Hjermann, I. Holme, and P. Urdal. "Lifestyle Changes May Reverse Development of the Insulin Resistance Syndrome. The Oslo Diet and Exercise Study: a Randomized Trial." *Diabetes Care* 20, no. 1 (January 1, 1997): 26–31.

"Trans Fatty Acids and Heart Disease > Publications > ACSH", n.d. http://www.acsh.org/publications/pubid.1415/pub_detail.asp.

"Type 1 - American Diabetes Association", n.d. http://www.diabetes.org/diabetes-basics/type-1/? loc=DropDownDB-type1.

La Vecchia, C., E Negri, and S. Franceschi. "A Case-control Study of Diabetes Mellitus and Cancer Risk." *British Journal of Cancer* 70 (1994): 950–953.

Velussi, M, AM Cernigoi, AD Monte, and etal. "Long-term (12 Months) Treatment with an Anti-oxidant Drug (silymarin) Is Effective on Hyperinsulinemia, Exogenous Insulin Need and Malondialdehyde Levels in Cirrhotic Diabetic Patients." *Journal of Hepatology* 26 (1997): 871–879.

Weatherby, Dicken. *Insider's Guide to the Functional Physiology of the Adrenal Glands*. Oregon: Weatherby and Associates, 2010.

Writing Group Members, Véronique L. Roger, Alan S. Go, Donald M. Lloyd-Jones, Emelia J. Benjamin, Jarett D. Berry, William B. Borden, et al. "Heart Disease and Stroke Statistics—2012 Update." *Circulation* 125, no. 1 (January 3, 2012): e2 –e220.

Yu, Herbert, and Thomas Rohan. "Role of the Insulin-Like Growth Factor Family in Cancer Development and Progression." *Journal of the National Cancer Institute* 92, no. 18 (September 20, 2000): 1472 –1489.

Made in the USA
Charleston, SC
18 October 2012